HOLGER VORNHOLT

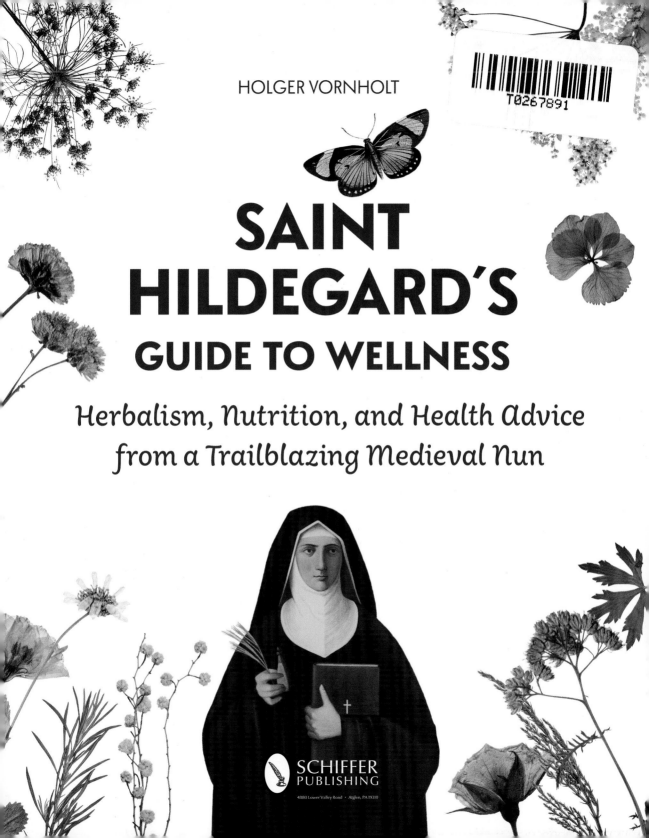

SAINT HILDEGARD'S
GUIDE TO WELLNESS

Herbalism, Nutrition, and Health Advice
from a Trailblazing Medieval Nun

SCHIFFER
PUBLISHING

4880 Lower Valley Road · Atglen, PA 19310

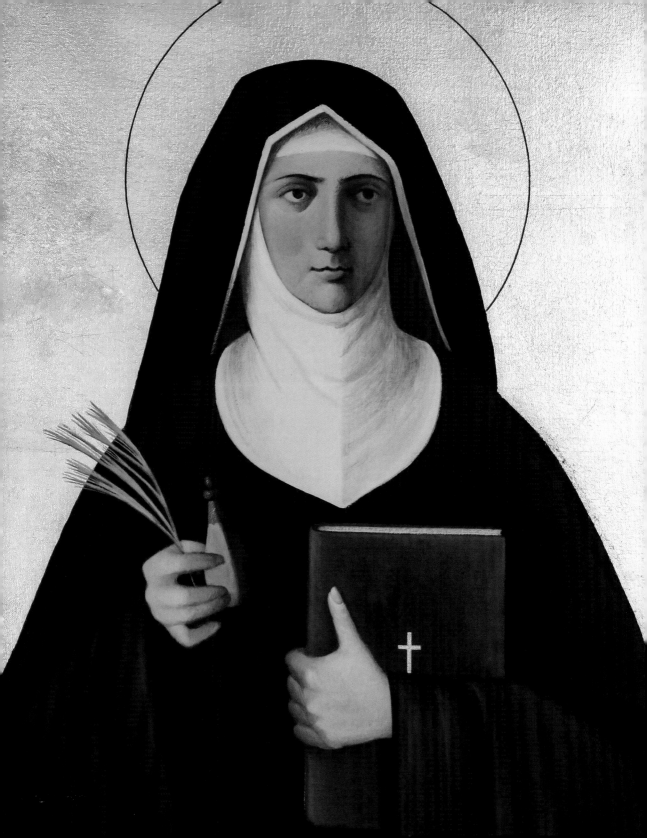

FOREWORD

An eminent abbess, poet, and composer, Hildegard of Bingen ranks as one of the most iconic female personalities of the Middle Ages. Even though she, as a woman, had no access to a classical medieval academic education, she made a name for herself as a universal scholar through her works on natural science and medicine. Within the Catholic Church, she is one of the four women—alongside Teresa of Ávila, Thérèse of Lisieux, and Catherine of Siena—who are revered not only as saints but also as doctors of the church.

It is for her writings on natural medicine that Hildegard is chiefly remembered among the general public today. These long-lost documents were rediscovered after 1950 by the Austrian physician Dr. Gottfried Hertzka, and Hildegard's medical and therapeutic knowledge was found to be still highly relevant in many respects, particularly jelling with the findings of modern nutritional physiology. A healthful diet is central to Hildegardian medicine. In all, Hildegard of Bingen described and studied the human health benefits of more than two hundred plants. And although she did this using the—by today's standards—primitive and unscientific methods of the High Middle Ages, some of her insights remain more valid today than ever.

Hildegard's medicine places great emphasis on medicinal herbs, which is not surprising given that herbs were the only effective "medicine" available in the Middle Ages. Any assessment of their medical efficacy should, however, take into account the circumstances of Hildegard's life and her spiritual background, according to which godly behavior was just as important as medication for the treatment of disease and the maintenance of general health. Nevertheless, many of the herbal healing effects described by Hildegard are corroborated by modern science. Conversely, she was not aware of potentially harmful effects of certain plants, especially for pregnant women, or of individual allergic and hypersensitive reactions. Therefore, Hildegard's herbs should be used only in a complementary capacity and never as a straight substitute for medical diagnosis and treatment.

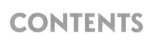

CONTENTS

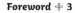

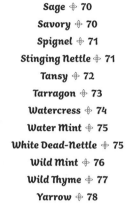

7.
HILDEGARD'S FAVORITE HERBS FROM A TO Z

8.
HILDEGARD'S HERBAL COSMETICS

9.
HILDEGARD OF BINGEN AND GEMSTONES

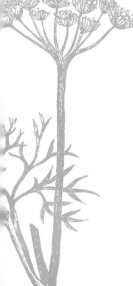

1.

WHO WAS
HILDEGARD OF BINGEN?

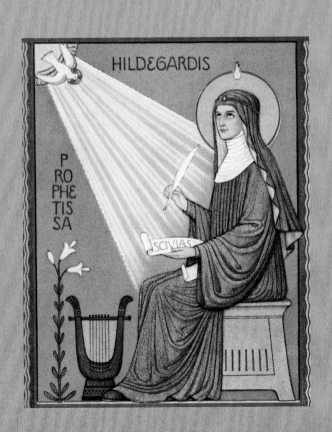

ildegard of Bingen was born in 1098 near Alzey in the German Rhineland, as the tenth child of the nobleman Hildebert of Bermersheim and his wife, Mechthild. She was born into an era when the Crusaders were attempting to take the Holy Land from the Arabs and the conflict between empire and papacy in Europe was at its height. From the moment of Hildegard's birth, her parents were determined that their child would lead a religious life, by way of a "tithe" to God. Her exceptionally keen interest in her environment was noticeable from her infancy, and she astonished her parents by experiencing her first visions at the age of three. On November 1, 1106, at the age of eight, she was sent to Disibodenberg Monastery, where she was placed under the tutelage of Jutta von Sponheim. Jutta took Hildegard into her anchorite's cell to prepare Hildegard for her vocation, which she assumed sometime between 1112 and 1115, taking her vows as a Benedictine nun.

At Disibodenberg

Over the following years, Hildegard was educated in the virtues and in music, although as a woman she was denied access to the medieval sciences. Officially, therefore, she was regarded throughout her lifetime as "untaught." Despite this, she acquired—at her own initiative and with the support of her confessor, Volmar—a wealth of knowledge that she supplemented with her own observations and whose breadth is quite astonishing even by modern standards.

In 1136, Jutta von Sponheim died and a new abbess had to be found for the monastery she had led for three decades. Hildegard was chosen, and—after some reflection—she eventually accepted the role. Just five years later, in 1141, Hildegard began to experience her famous visions, which she documented, with Volmar's assistance, in her work Scivias. The title comes from the Latin phrase sci vias, meaning "know the ways." The work created quite a stir, attracting the attention of such august figures as

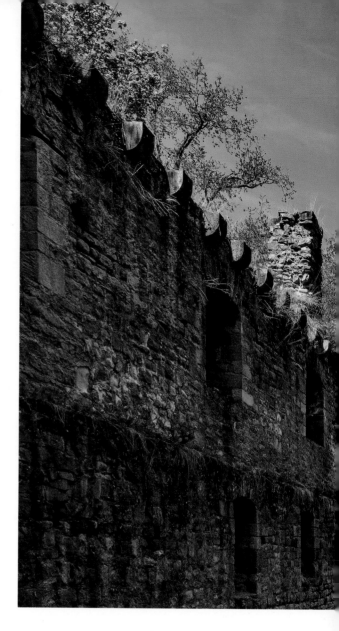

Pope Eugene III and St. Bernard of Clairvaux. Strictly speaking, women were not allowed to write books at that time, but from then on, Hildegard was authorized by the pope to use the official title of prophetess. She was a magnet that attracted young people who flocked to Disibodenberg until the monastery began to burst at the seams.

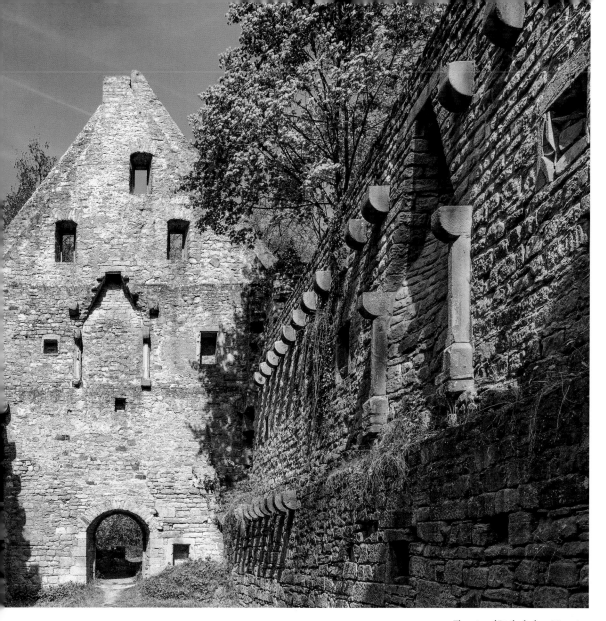

The ruins of Disibodenberg Monastery

In 1150, despite many difficulties, she eventually succeeded in founding a new convent at Rupertsberg, which was funded by gifts from noble families. Hildegard became abbess, and after a long search, she finally managed to secure the preeminent Emperor Frederick Barbarossa as secular patron.

Writings on Natural Science

Hildegard's second major work, *The Book of Subtleties of the Diverse Nature of Things*, was written between 1151 and 1158. The first part—titled *Physica*—was a comprehensive natural history containing descriptions of numerous animals and plants, along with early references to the healing powers of certain plants. In the second part of the work, she set out her medical knowledge. The book, *Causae et Curae* ("Causes and Cures"), remains highly relevant to this day in its holistic approach to mind and body, and it still holds the key to many a mystery. While the main emphasis of Hildegard's medicine was on healing herbs, she used other plants to treat diseases too and described the curative effects of fruit trees— apple, quince, pear, cherry, apricot, plum, birch, chestnut, and elder—as well as those of more exotic plants such as aloe vera, galangal, and ginger. Grains—particularly spelt, oats, and rye—also had their place in her medicine chest.

The Final Years

Thanks to Hildegard's enduring appeal, her community soon outgrew the Rupertsberg Monastery, prompting her to found Eibingen Abbey in 1165. By then, she was approaching seventy years old, which was quite an advanced age in the medieval era. Between 1160 and 1170, she also accomplished the great feat of completing four extensive preaching tours that took her across southern Germany and well into France.

In 1173, Hildegard's confessor and secretary Volmar died—a bitter blow to Hildegard after their almost sixty years of cooperation. He was not survived long by his successor, Gottfried, a monk from Disibodenberg Monastery, who died in 1176. The new incumbent was Wibert of Gembloux, who accompanied the now-almost-eighty-year-old nun through her last months. On September 17, 1179, Hildegard finally passed away at age eighty-one at Rupertsberg Monastery.

Hildegard's work, however, has lived on for centuries—particularly her nutritional theory, which anticipated many modern approaches and transmitted a wealth of knowledge that took another 850 years to be scientifically proven. As for her writings on natural science and her music, they too are timeless and still rank today among the "jewels" of the medieval period.

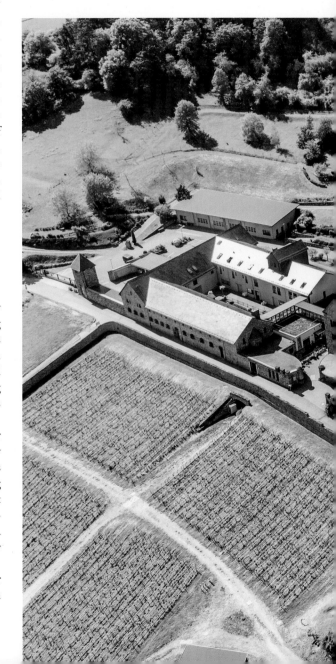

The Benedictine Abbey of St. Hildegard on the site of Eibingen Monastery

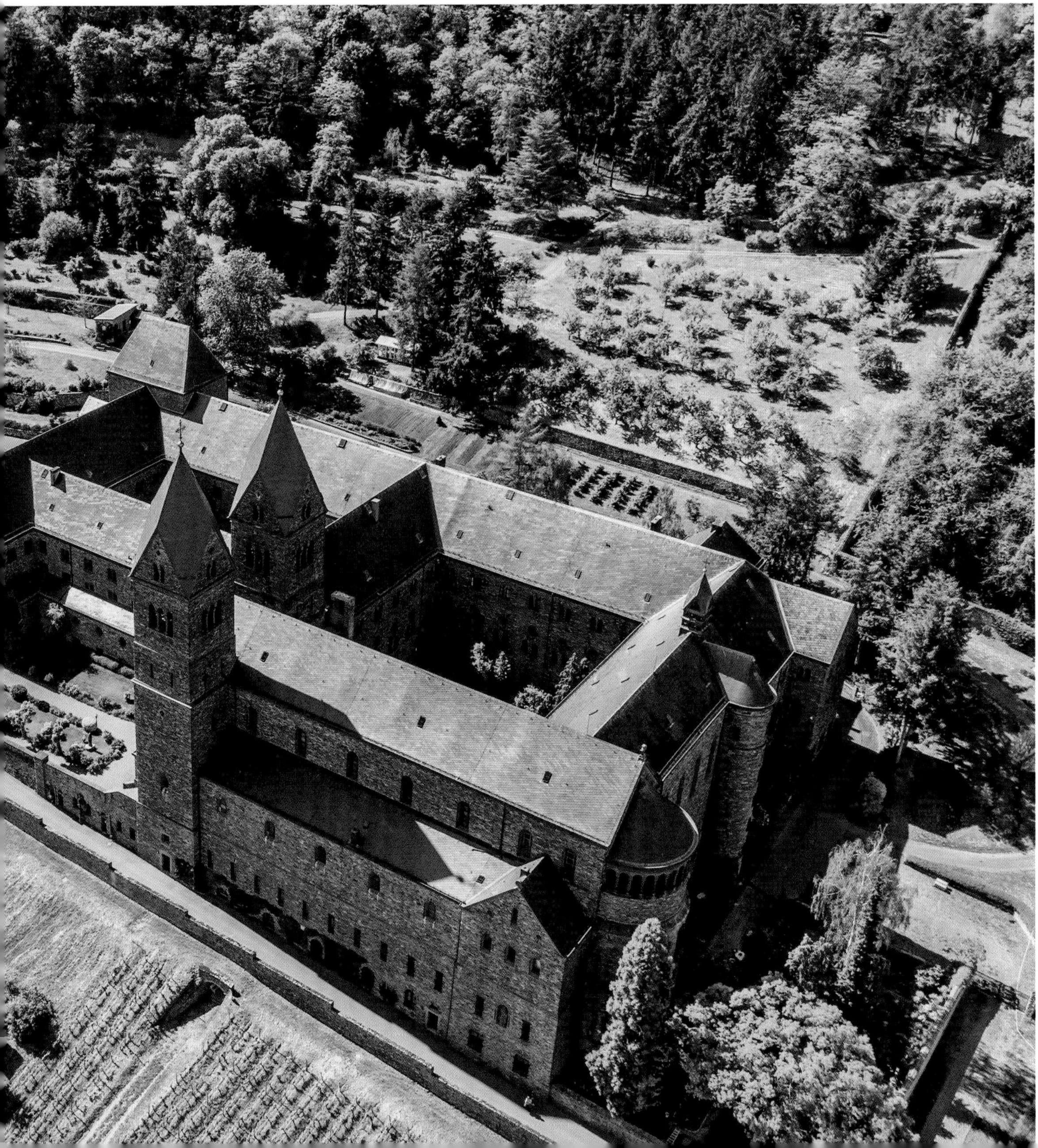

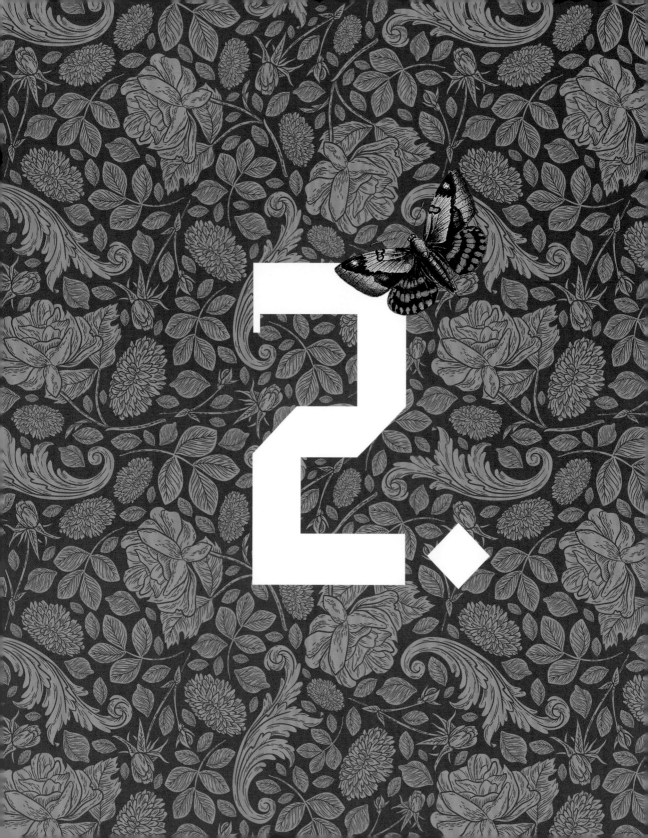

2.

HEALTHFUL NUTRITION FOR A HEALTHY BODY AND MIND

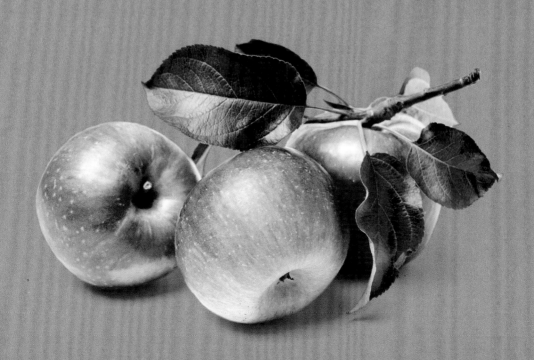

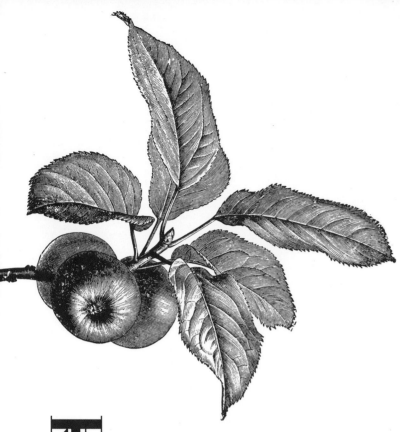

The development of humanity—from the first primitive nomadic societies, through the flourishing prehistoric and ancient civilizations, to affluent modern societies—is inextricably bound up with the development of its dietary habits. Indeed, regarded as one of our species' greatest cultural achievements is humanity's transition from being nomadic hunter-gatherers—following the migrations of large herds of foraging cattle year after year—into establishing the first settled farming societies.

Hunter-Gatherers

This step was accompanied by a change in diet. Or rather vice versa: the desire for a better diet was, in all likelihood, a key motivation for settling. As hunter-gatherers, humans lived on their quarry along with fish and the fruits and nuts they happened upon during their foraging expeditions. Even after settling down, they could still scour the area around their new settlements for nature's edible treasures and bring them home, but something new and unfamiliar had also entered their lives that would bring about a radical change in their nutrition: the practice of grain and vegetable cultivation.

The "Invention" of Grain

All ancient civilizations were based on the cultivation and trading of grain: the Sumerians, Babylonians, and Assyrians in the Mesopotamian basin between the Euphrates and the Tigris; the Phrygians, Lydians, and Hittites in Asia Minor; the Minoans on Crete; the different kingdoms of ancient Egypt; and later the Greek city-states and the emergent Roman Republic. Livestock farming was far less developed than it is today, and the main foodstuffs were grain, fruit, and vegetables. The grain was not yet used to make bread, however, but mostly gruel. Baked bread came later and was initially regarded as the food of the rich. The proportion of plant-based food was much higher 2,000–3,000 years ago than nowadays, and that of animal products accordingly lower.

Intemperance and Health

During the first few centuries of the Common Era, a process of mental, cultural, economic, political, and military decline set in in the post-Republican Roman Empire, which is nowadays often characterized as the period of "decadence." This decline extended to dietary habits and thus had a direct impact on public health. Healthful moderation gave way to intemperance, feasting, and gluttony. How far this process—also described by Roman authors of the time—contributed to the downfall of the Roman Empire is open to question, but it seems certain that the new eating habits combined with rapidly increasing alcohol consumption to lead to a sudden rise in diet-related diseases.

The Consequences of Poor Diet

Poor diet still has fatal consequences today. Modern humans lead a lifestyle of abundance, eating much more than our ancestors from past millennia yet often using far less energy due to a lack of physical exercise. The consequences are obesity, metabolic or cardiovascular diseases, and many other health problems. In the US, some medical experts now attribute around two-thirds of all deaths to bad diet. Nutritionally worthless foods with too much animal protein, fat, and salt along with refined flour and industrial sugar are the target of particular criticism from many nutritional scientists, who advocate replacing such foods with a simple wholefood diet of grains, fruit, and vegetables. In this respect, the nutritional theory developed by Hildegard over eight hundred years ago is perhaps more timely than ever. It harks back to the natural foods of her day, many of which have been forgotten or sidelined—if not entirely displaced—by ones that are more "modern" and profitable. And even in the case of foods that may have been as popular in the High Middle Ages as they are today (such as certain types of fruit, for instance), the original varieties have been overwhelmingly replaced by standardized, industrially grown, and processed strains.

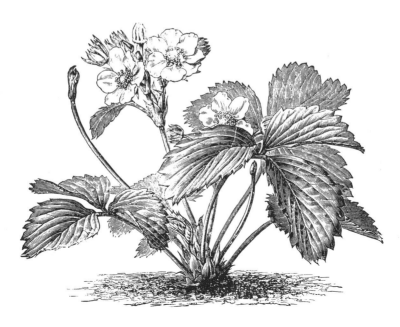

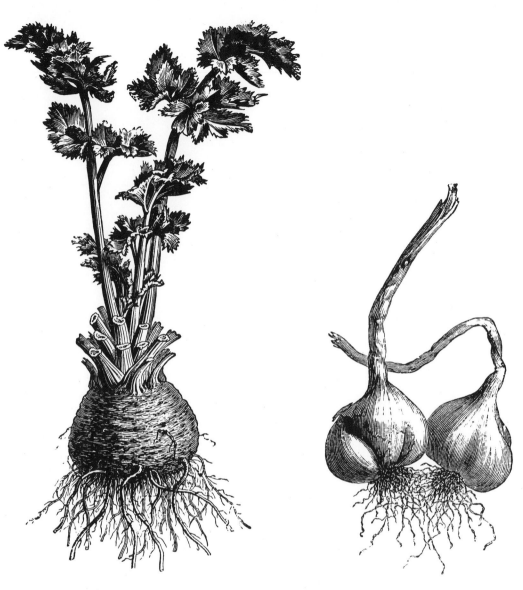

Hildegard's Nutritional Therapy

Hildegard of Bingen's nutritional therapy is essentially based on spelt, a special type of grain that lends itself both to baking and boiling. Her approach is a holistic one, however—no food group is categorically condemned. Besides the positive properties of spelt, she also notes the health benefits of eating fruit and vegetables, as well as moderate amounts of fish, meat, and liver. Complementing these are the all-important medicinal herbs. The results are quite remarkable: a dietary plan based on Hildegard's teaching can prevent most nutritionally related diseases. Moreover, there is nothing "bitter" about this medicine. On the contrary, the recipes from Hildegard's kitchen are invariably found to be exceptionally tasty, so much so that many individuals and their families tend to stick with them for a lifetime.

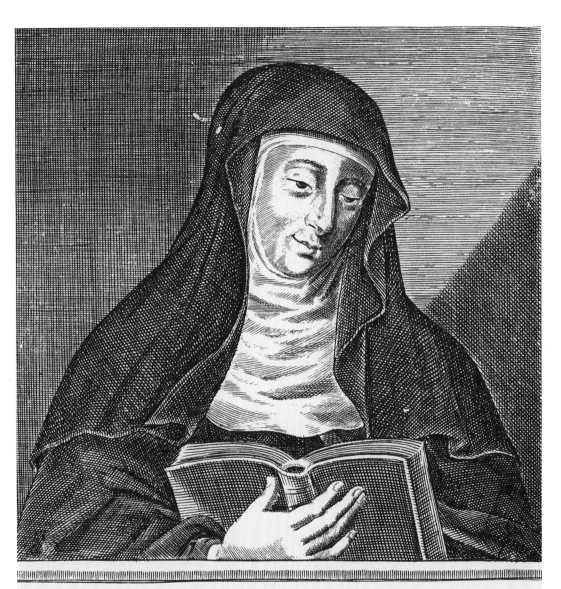

HILDE GARDIS *a Virgin Prophetess,* Abbeſs of
Sᵗ *Rvperts Nunnerye. She died at Bingen* Aᵒ Do:
1180. *Aged* 82 *yeares.*

all ſc:l

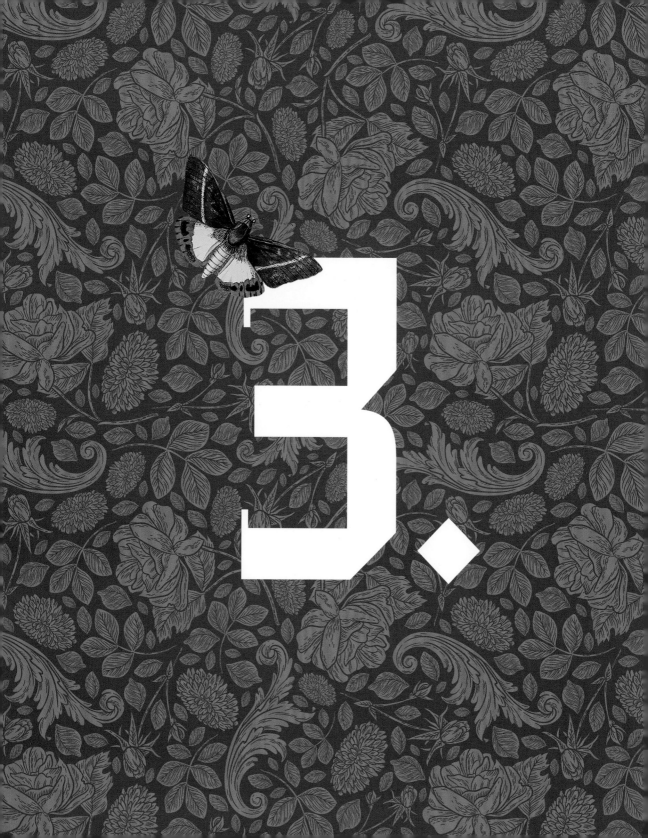

3.

WHY IS
HILDEGARD OF BINGEN
STILL SO RELEVANT TODAY?

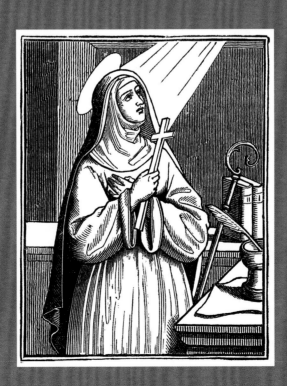

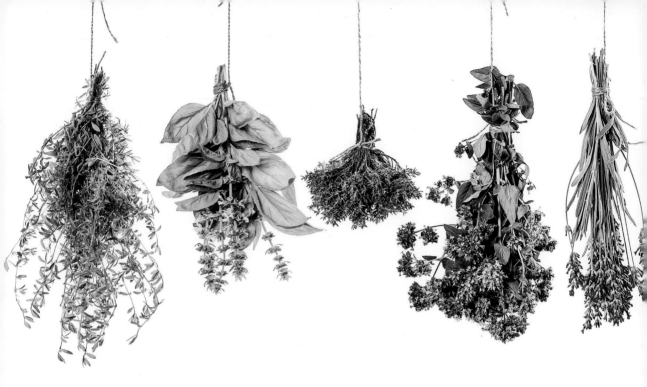

ritics may question why Hildegard of Bingen's health and nutrition program remains so timelessly relevant more than eight hundred years on. The answer is quite simple: as a holistic concept, it doesn't just promote a healthful diet for its own sake, but it's part of a strategy whereby a healthful lifestyle is understood as the foundation for mental health—true to the ancient motto "mens sana in corpore sano," or "a healthy mind in a healthy body." The merits of this approach were already recognized during Hildegard's own lifetime; it's no wonder she was a sought-after advisor to emperors, kings, popes, and other spiritual and secular leaders. Thanks to the rediscovery of her writings, Hildegard's knowledge is now accessible to all sectors of society, and—given the current state of public health—it is perhaps more pertinent than ever. Nowhere else do we find such sophisticated and detailed descriptions of the curative powers of specific foodstuffs. As such, her brand of medicine is groundbreaking and unparalleled in our cultural sphere. Its importance is equal to that of

the great medical theories of Far Eastern cultures. Plus, it has the added advantage of being all encompassing, so that anyone following Hildegard's recipes need follow no other diet and can dispense with calorie tables.

The strength of this approach lies in its firm reliance on nature and its riches, which offer everything we modern humans need for a healthy life.

Countering the Diseases of Civilization

It no longer comes as a surprise to anyone when nutritional scientists publish research showing that a balanced diet can prevent a number of the so-called diseases of civilization, including some types of cancer. What is astonishing, however, is the fact that Hildegard of Bingen recognized and documented this fact more than 850 years ago and bequeathed us a nutritional

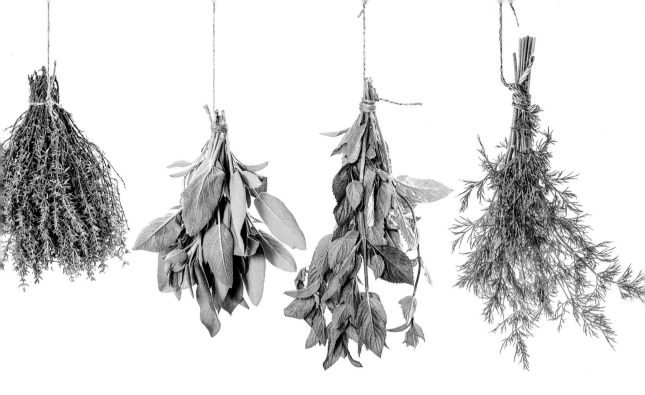

therapy based on spelt, fruit, vegetables, and medicinal herbs that offers protection against many diseases. The important thing is to choose the right foods, since not all will guarantee an equally healthful diet. Hildegard makes a very clear distinction between "healthful" foods, which are foods that have neither a positive nor a negative impact on health, and "unhealthful" foods, which can make us ill if consumed persistently or to excess. Specifically, the Hildegard diet comprises a varied range of whole foods with spelt, fruit, and vegetables at its core and meat and dairy as a welcome but sparingly used adjunct. Needless to say, Hildegard had no access to analytical data on nutrients, vitamins, trace elements, or calories; she classified foods according to their curative value for the human body. This makes it all the more remarkable that her theories have been broadly confirmed by modern food chemistry research and can thus claim scientific support.

Of course, a medical book from the High Middle Ages was never written with the twenty-first century in mind. Hildegard's research and treatises related to her own era and constituted a general investigation into the healing power of a natural diet and its medicinal effects. Her findings are assembled in the nine books of her work *Physica* and the medical textbook *Causae et Curae*, on the causes of and possible treatments for various diseases. For centuries, these works languished in obscurity until their rediscovery in the second half of the twentieth century. Dr. Gottfried Herzka, from the southern German city of Konstanz, was the first to apply Hildegard's nutritional therapy to modern times and systematically put her guidelines into practice. Since then, Hildegard of Bingen's nutritional theory has helped thousands of people who had been suffering for years from the consequences of poor diet.

Basic Principles for a Healthy Life

On the basis of her religious understanding, Hildegard of Bingen formulated six basic principles that she considered crucial to a generally healthful lifestyle. These relate to the metaphysical sphere and extend far beyond nutrition. Every human being, she believed, has a duty to follow these basic rules of life in a spirit of mental and physical self-determination. This is the key to maintaining or restoring good health. First, she urges great care in selecting the right foods for our daily needs. Second, she exhorts all human beings to live in harmony with nature and the universe. Next, we must find the right balance between exercise and rest, prayer and meditation. Similar moderation should be observed in terms of sleeping and waking, in order to bring strained nerves into equilibrium. Overeating should likewise be avoided; rather, we should take care to cleanse the body of toxins and waste products. Finally, Hildegard encourages every individual to transform fear, anxiety, and distress into positive energy—what we would now call "positive thinking." This helps boost both our mental health and our immune system. Once again, these guidelines are highly relevant to our own age: in our affluent society, where food has increasingly come to be regarded as a status symbol and demonstration of economic prosperity, the very stuff that is meant to sustain us has become a major cause of illness. Thus, allergies, arteriosclerosis, autoimmune disorders, diabetes, heart disease, cancer, cirrhosis of the liver, and stroke now top the list of serious diseases.

Hildegard's Golden Rules at a Glance

❋ Take great care to select the right foods for daily consumption.
❋ Live in harmony with the universe and nature.
❋ Maintain a balance among rest, meditation, prayer, and exercise.
❋ Don't sleep too much—or too little!
❋ Avoid overeating and detoxify the body regularly.
❋ Positive thinking: transform fear and anxiety into positive energy.

Combating Stress with Positive Vitality

A healthful diet alone cannot guarantee human health if all the other key factors are neglected, however. This applies in particular to the body's vital recovery phase—namely, sleep. In our modern performance- and leisure-oriented society, human beings are exposed to constant stress. In order to ensure a sensible balance among performance, work, and leisure, we must draw on complementary forms of energy. According to Hildegard, there are thirty-five vital energies that must be actively reconciled in order to lead a contented, fulfilled, and self-determined life. These include love and inner strength, as well as the art of being happy. Hildegard calls for the performance-oriented existence

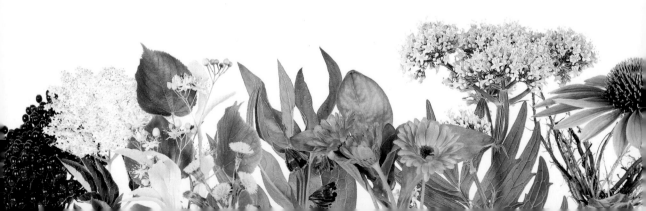

to be balanced with a spiritual and creative existence, consisting of a certain introspection that can be achieved either through meditation or through walking and other activities. To do this, however, we need to recharge regularly through restorative sleep.

Only sleep can regenerate body and mind so that both remain equal to the constant demands of everyday life. Thus, sleep—and, in particular, dreaming—is highly important for performance, as anyone who has ever struggled out of bed after a haunted night will confirm. To promote restful sleep with pleasant dreams, before one goes to bed, Hildegard recommends a cup of orange blossom tea, 1–2 tablespoons of poppy seeds in apple compote, or both; a lavender bath; and, finally, a good book. For good measure, one should use a pillow stuffed with the herb betony and place a jasper stone on the skin close to the heart at night. As a general aid to healthful sleep, one should go for a walk in the fresh air and in beautiful surroundings for at least an hour every day. Other forms of exercise and hobbies such as running, cycling, swimming, dancing, and so on are also ideal. What's more, they help burn calories and so prevent obesity and, ultimately, sickness. Last but not least, all these activities strengthen the immune system, help relieve stress and promote inner calm, stimulate the metabolism, and improve performance.

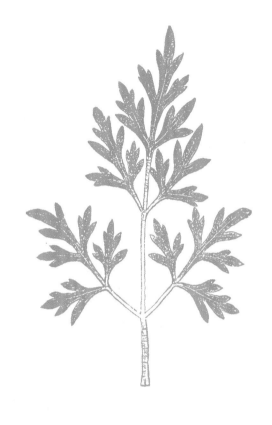

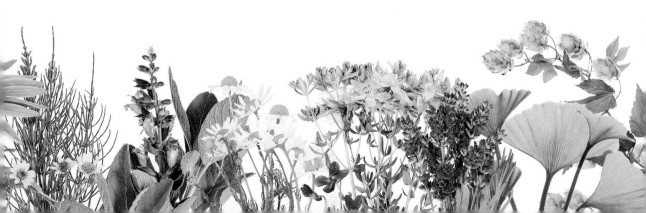

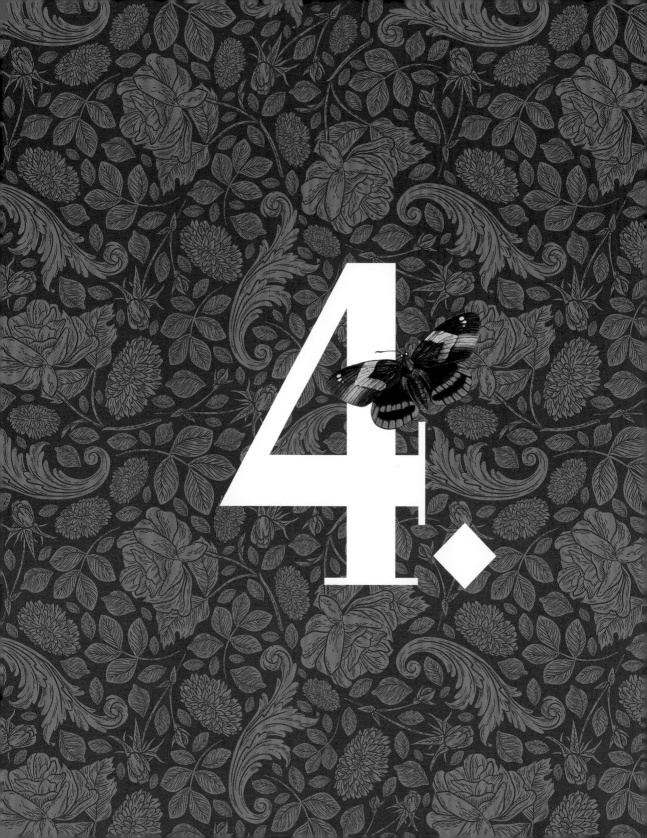

4.

HILDEGARD AND
THE HUMAN BODY

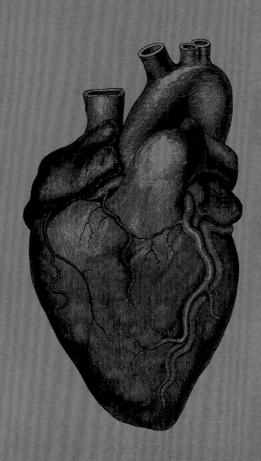

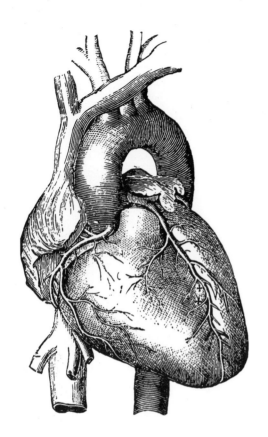

The Cardiovascular System

Diseases of the cardiovascular system are the number one killer in our affluent society. Many people will be diagnosed at least once during their lifetime with obesity, high blood pressure, arteriosclerosis, angina, or high cholesterol, for example. Added to these are the problems of permanent emotional, mental, and physical overload—not to mention the sensory overload caused by a seemingly ever-accelerating world and the lure of stimulants such as nicotine, alcohol, and drugs. In Hildegardian medicine, cardiovascular diseases are traced to several basic causes.

A large proportion of cardiovascular patients are from "cardiac families" with a disposition toward this type of disease. Another large share of cases are the result of poor diet and lifestyle: too much of the wrong kinds of food, especially fatty foods, and excessive smoking and drinking. The third risk factor, which should not be underestimated, is a psychological one. In many people, constant stress, irresolvable unhappiness, and other emotional stresses impact more or less directly on an often already weakened heart.

Digestion Part 1: The Stomach

The digestion of food is of crucial importance to Hildegard, and she places special emphasis on the stomach as the first stage in the passage of food through the human body. In her view, overeating and poor diet are the main causes of gastric complaints. She is particularly critical of the raw foods so popular today, on the grounds that their digestion takes too much energy out of the body and that they can putrefy if processed too slowly: "People sometimes consume foods to excess, and these cannot be processed in the stomach because they were eaten raw or uncooked or only half cooked. This food hardens in the stomach, and the person becomes ill." To aid gastric digestion, Hildegard recommends drinking plenty of fluid with meals. It is here too that her preference for spelt first comes into play, as a substance that is easily broken down without too much digestive effort, thereby releasing all its vital nutrients and vitamins into the body.

F or Hildegard, human health depended above all on nutrition. Her knowledge of the biological value of the many foods available to us, the healing powers she attributed to them, and their practical use in her recipes are a great help to modern humans when it comes to adopting a sensible lifestyle and eating healthfully, sustainably, and in harmony with nature. The following chapter considers which parts of the human body are most at risk in today's hectic, stressful world; how harmful environmental influences affect us in different phases of life; and what difference can be made by lifestyle choices.

Digestion Part 2: The Gut

The gut—being the most important element of the digestive system, even more so than the stomach—is central to Hildegard's medical theory. Indeed, she traces almost all illnesses back to this organ. Particular importance is attached to the health of the intestinal flora, as a vital prerequisite for healthful digestion. As in the case of cardiovascular diseases, damage to these useful microorganisms is often caused by poor diet and partly also by a stressful lifestyle.

Unfortunately, some of the drugs prescribed nowadays also destroy the intestinal flora, thereby causing a variety of diseases that they are actually designed to cure. This problem is compounded by numerous pollutants in our food such as heavy metals and pesticide residues, as well as food additives such as sweeteners or preservatives, which can be the final straw for an already weakened gut. The consequences are often stubborn diarrheal diseases with spasmodic flatulence and sometimes also sluggish bowel movements and constipation. For this reason, Hildegard almost invariably prescribes a thorough cleansing of the intestinal flora by means of a spelt diet prior to treating any other illness. Longer-term, persistent, and chronic diarrheal diseases in particular demand patience and cannot be cured from one day to the next. It can easily take up to six months for the digestion to normalize again. In Hildegardian medicine, the chances of curing diarrhea with an anti-inflammatory, fiber-rich, and flour-rich spelt diet are estimated at 90 percent. As a first step, the digestive system has to adjust to spelt and gradually get used to it. The success of this approach depends on the use of pure spelt that has not been crossbred with wheat or polluted with agrochemical residues.

The Body's Chemical Factory: The Liver

The liver is the body's chemical factory, and it fulfills a whole range of important functions simultaneously without us even noticing—as long as it is healthy. Diseases of the liver, like those of the cardiovascular and digestive systems, are often caused by lifestyle factors: eating and drinking too much, eating and drinking the wrong things, and high levels of stress that prevent us from processing our emotions, particularly the negative ones. Hildegard herself observes, "If one consumes all foods without moderation and abstinence, this can cause the liver to become damaged and enlarged, and the juices it sends to all the organs to be destroyed." And it is true that overloading the liver with the toxins contained in food or pharmaceuticals and the waste products generated by a bad diet, exposing it to toxic metabolic products, and subjecting it to the effects of alcohol and drugs can cause it to become swollen and effectively blocked. In such cases, the only remedy is indeed to switch to a conscious lifestyle and diet and abstain from all known liver toxins.

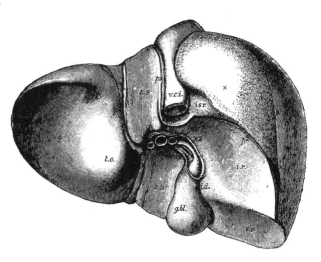

The Seat of the Emotions: The Gallbladder

Most incidences of liver stress and disease are inextricably linked to similar processes in the gallbladder. Here too, Hildegard identifies the irresponsible consumption of foods and stimulants and an unbalanced emotional life as the main causes of illness. This results in a pathogenic overproduction of bile acid, which is released into the gut, where it causes further damage. Hildegard calls this excess acid "black bile." In her view, the right amount of bile acid is also key to a person's character traits: "A person whose black bile is very strong is easily moved to anger. Such a person is prone to sudden and violent outbursts of rage." She knew the solution to this problem already, however: "Black bile decreases with good, tasty foods and increases with bad, bitter, unclean, and poorly prepared foods." Once again, she recommends spelt to calm the inflamed gallbladder and restore it to health. Today, we know that bile acid and cholesterol levels are closely linked.

The Gateway to the Outside World: The Lungs

Generally speaking, diseases of the lungs were undoubtedly a bigger problem in Hildegard's time than today. Nevertheless, large numbers of people still die of conditions such as pneumonia, tuberculosis, or lung cancer. Hildegardian medicine identifies three main causes of lung disease. As with heart disease, many lung conditions also have a genetic component. And as with nearly all diseases, those of the lung and upper respiratory tract are also affected by a person's emotional state and morale. Finally, the lungs—as the "gateway" connecting us directly to the outside world every second of our sleeping or waking lives—are particularly vulnerable to the pollutants absorbed with the air we breathe. Nowadays, these may consist of involuntarily inhaled pathogens and harmful toxins from traffic, industry, and agriculture. Another major source of harm is the voluntarily inhaled cocktail of toxins contained in cigarette smoke.

The Body's Waste Treatment System: The Kidneys

If the liver is the body's chemical factory, then the kidneys can be aptly described as its waste disposal system. Round the clock, day in, day out, they filter the blood, extract urine, remove waste products, and regulate the body's fluid balance. If the kidney function is impaired, this can lead to high blood pressure and edema. It also increases the risk of kidney stones, which can be painful, particularly if caused by a concentration of certain substances; almost two-thirds of all kidney stones are attributable to excessive levels of oxalic acid in food, for example. The omnipresence of stress is probably also a factor. Other common causes are an oversaturation of uric acid due to excessive meat and alcohol consumption. Besides stress reduction, the best way to avoid kidney stones is to cut out milk and dairy products, meat, chard and spinach, cocoa and chocolate, and coffee and black tea. Above all, it is essential to drink at least 2 liters (about a half gallon) of water and other fluids a day.

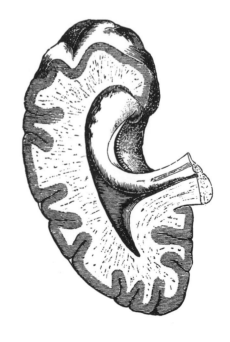

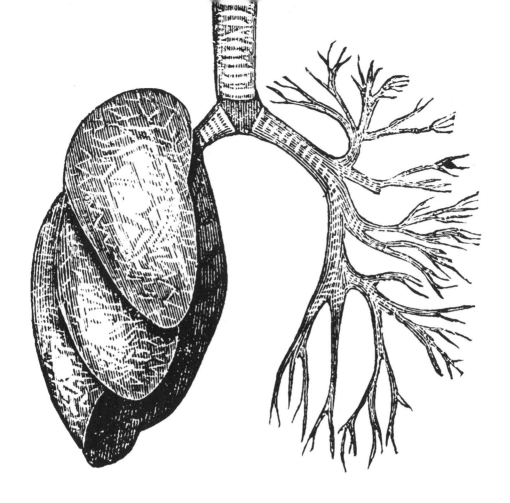

The Elixir of Life: The Blood

A common disease of the blood is anemia, and its symptoms include pallor and general weakness. It is caused by a lack of iron, which is responsible for building the red pigment of the blood needed to transport oxygen around the body and so ensure its general vitality. To counter iron deficiency, Hildegard recommends the consumption of animal liver, which is known to be particularly rich in iron. This type of iron has a higher bioavailability than the pharmaceutical variety in standard iron tablets, meaning that it is much more easily absorbed and metabolized by the human body. Hildegard's preferred source is chicken liver: "The liver of a chicken is good to eat against all infirmities that harm a person internally." The next best options are deer liver, cow and calf liver, lamb and goat liver, and—if nothing else is available—pig liver. At the same time, high liver consumption can also lead to high uric acid levels, causing gout in susceptible people. Nowadays, moreover, given the potential presence of residues of hormones, antibiotics, and other pollutants in slaughtered cattle, such foods should be treated with caution.

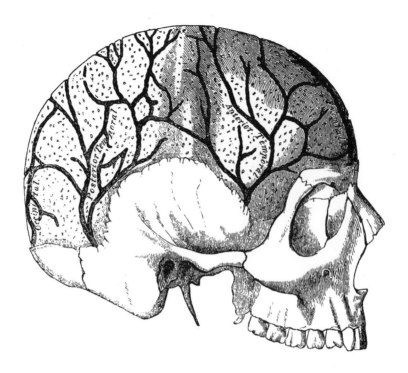

The Body's Stress Barometer: The Nervous System

According to Hildegard, "When a person feels that something is repugnant to his soul, the heart, liver, and gallbladder contract. This constriction releases a fog that hovers over the heart and darkens it, making the person feel sad." In other words, Hildegard considers the main causes of nervous disorders to be of an emotional nature, born of stress, fear, anxiety, frustration, and anger. Regardless of whether a person is more irritable or more prone to depression, the consequences are always illness-inducing. The most effective remedy in this case is to shut oneself off from the causes and find ways of avoiding them in the first place. To this end, we should strive to maintain a balanced overall constitution by getting plenty of restful sleep, occupying the mind with things we find pleasurable, and taking enough exercise.

The Body's Envelope: The Skin

Diseases of the skin are, sadly, extremely common nowadays. According to Hildegard's logic, they are—like most diseases—the result of an unhealthful diet and lifestyle. For this reason, Hildegardian medicine doesn't treat the skin directly but focuses on the gastrointestinal tract as well as the patient's external circumstances. The first step toward curing the problem is a thorough bowel cleanse, because poor diet is most visibly manifested on the skin. This is due to the accumulation of allergens in modern industrially processed foods, in some cases producing a veritable cocktail of toxins. Healthful alternatives include spelt and chestnut, if produced in a clean environment without the use of chemicals.

The Body's Scaffold: The Skeleton

Today, the most common diseases of the skeleton and particularly the joints are rheumatism and gout. Rheumatism in particular is not confined to the bones, however, but also affects the connective tissue and—in the advanced stages—the whole body. This disease is very hard to treat. Dietary changes based on Hildegard's principles are a good start, but they are often not enough. The aim in all cases is to rid the body as much as possible of toxic metabolic products and environmental poisons. By comparison, gout appears relatively easy to treat. It is caused by a persistently high level of uric acid in the blood; this then crystallizes in the joints, leading to very painful inflammations. The causes of gout are overconsumption of meat and other fatty and protein-rich foods, as well as overconsumption of wine. The risk of gout can be relatively easily eliminated, however, by switching to a Hildegard-style diet

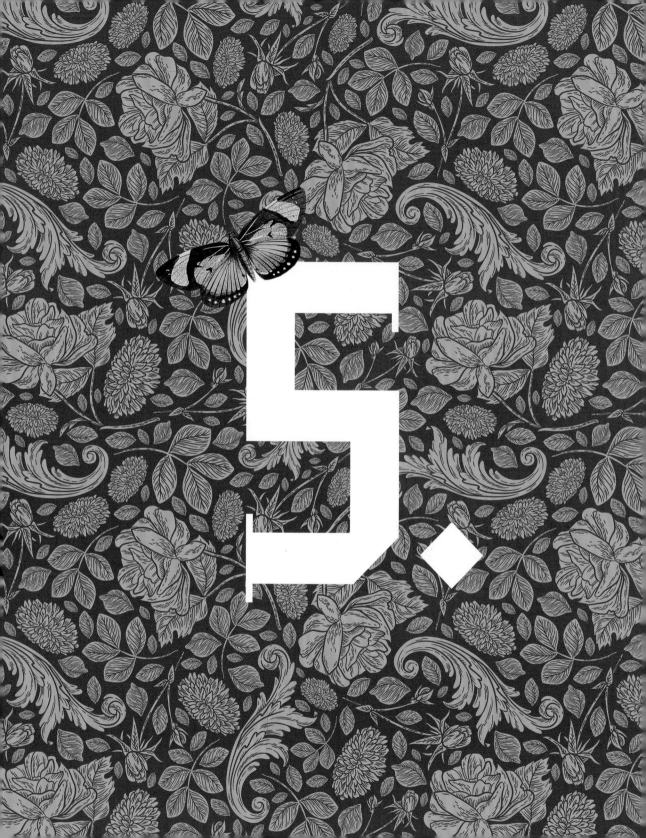

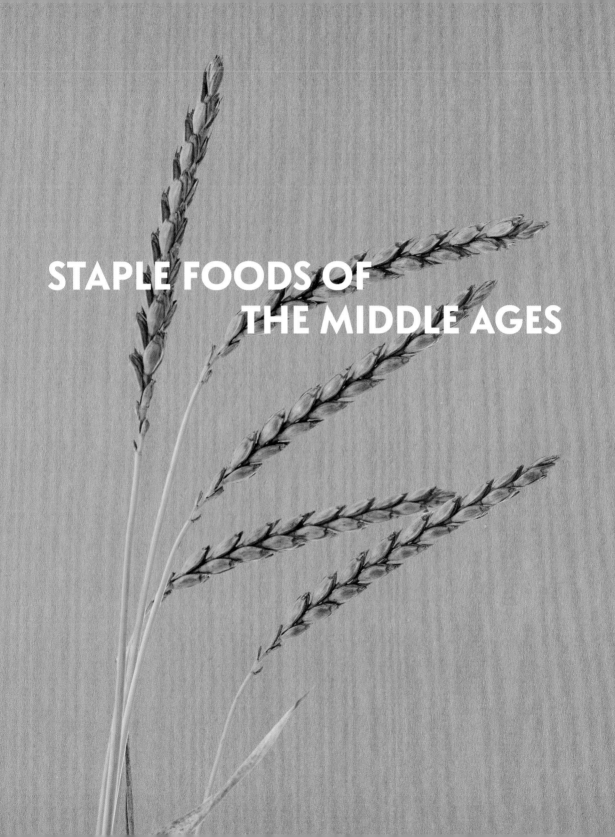

STAPLE FOODS OF
THE MIDDLE AGES

In medieval times, the overwhelming majority of the population relied on grain as the basis of their nutrition. In her work *Physica*, Hildegard of Bingen identifies spelt as the most valuable grain, and she indeed credits it with the greatest overall healing power of all foodstuffs. In second place are oats, which—although almost as effective as spelt—can occasionally lead to constipation. Next come rye and wheat; unlike spelt, however, these are pronounced totally unsuitable for cooking. Barley is not recommended for consumption by Hildegard due to a lack of healing power, and she explicitly advises against eating millet.

Hildegard of Bingen and Spelt

Spelt (*Triticum spelta*) is a variety of grain from the wheatgrass family and hence a relative of modern high-performance wheat varieties. Also known as dinkel wheat, spelt is a very ancient grain and one of the first grasses to have been domesticated by humans. It remained popular into the last century but has since been broadly displaced by wheat. Spelt is one of the most robust of all cereal crops. The grain is enclosed in a husk, which provides effective protection against

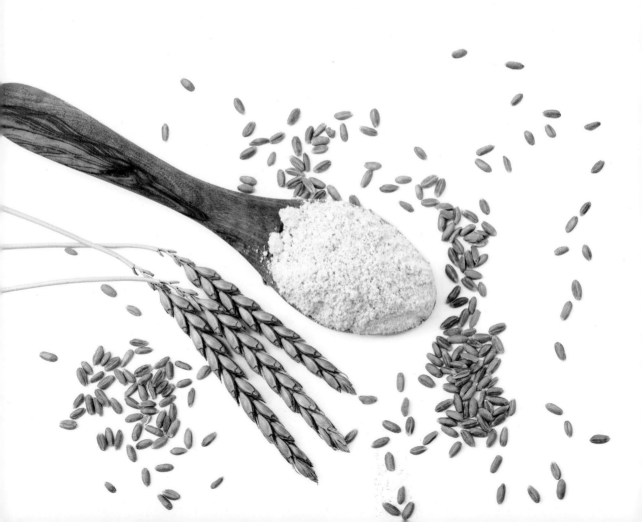

harmful environmental influences. This makes the plant relatively insensitive to weather conditions and less likely to absorb pollutants from the air. This low-maintenance cereal grain is very winter hardy and can be grown at altitudes of up to 3,281 feet (1,000 meters [m]). In addition, it can survive rainy periods and heatwaves alike without visible damage. As such, it is ideal for growing in extreme climates and yields acceptable harvests of consistent quality even in unfavorable conditions and scant soils. Spelt also has a low susceptibility to disease and needs little spraying. For this reason, it is generally much less polluted with pesticide residues than other types of grain. In contrast to wheat and rye, spelt also obviates the need for crop rotation since it absorbs fewer nutrients and places far less stress on the soil. Consequently, it can be planted in the same soil for several years in succession without adverse effects.

Spelt has a high protein content. Depending on local conditions and weather patterns, this can range between 10 and 18 percent—higher than in most wheat varieties. The vitamin and mineral content of spelt is also much higher than that of wheat, rye, and other grains. What's more, it is extremely gentle on the stomach and gut. This makes it easy to digest, resulting in a high level of bioavailability; in other words, the body is able to absorb all the goodness quickly and without loss. This improves the body's performance hugely in comparison to other types of grain. But it is not just for these reasons that spelt tops Hildegard's nutritional chart: it also contains other nutritional elements vital for sustaining human life. A crucial ingredient of spelt is rhodanide, which is important for the formation of stem cells in particular. Stem cells are what the body uses to make all other cells—whether nuclear, muscle, immune, blood, or nerve cells—so a spelt-based diet can be instrumental in promoting cell growth. Furthermore, rhodanide has antiallergic properties, which makes spelt suitable for treating food allergies. And last but not least, spelt helps prevent cancer, since rhodanide renders the cell walls impenetrable to carcinogenic substances.

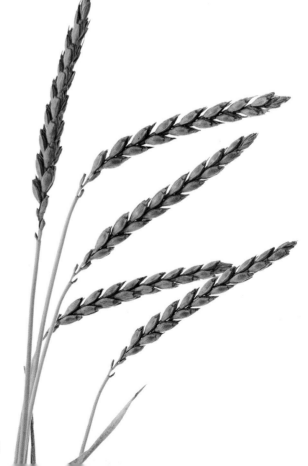

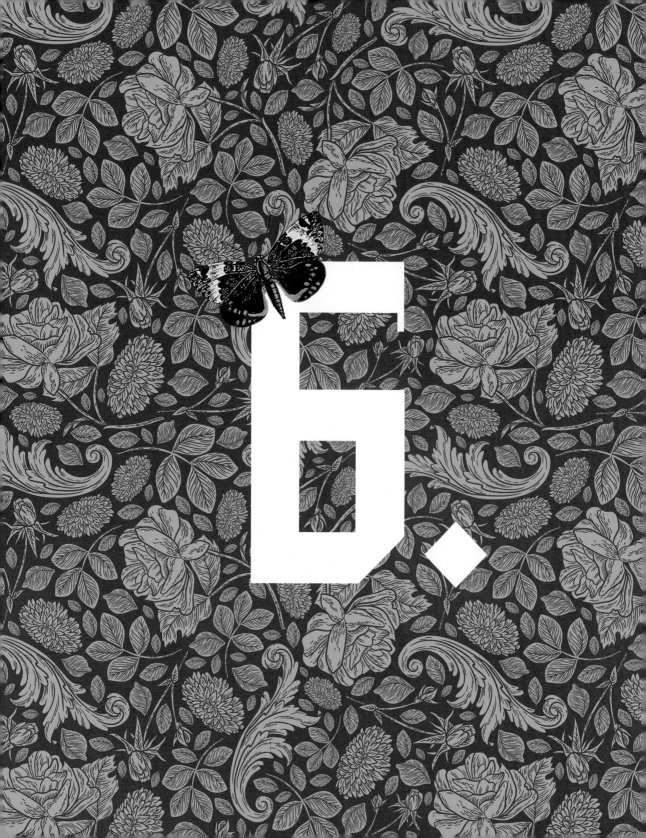

HILDEGARD OF BINGEN AND HERBS

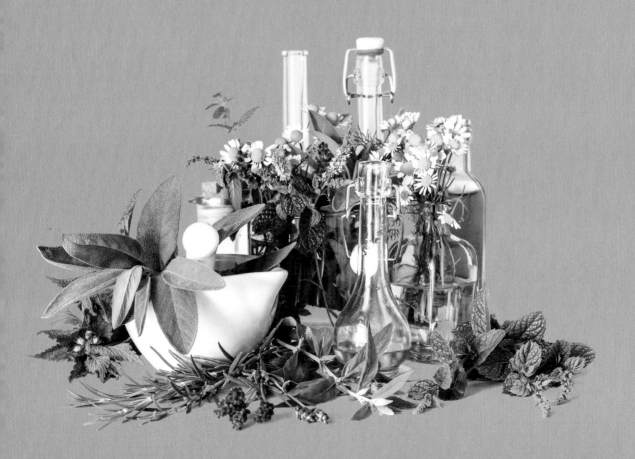

In accordance with the medical knowledge of the Middle Ages, Hildegard's medicine is based on the theory of the four humors. In this respect, she was perfectly up to date for her time, even though this theory dates back to late antiquity, originating in the second to the fifth centuries. The theory of the four humors was first formulated by the famous Greek physician Galen of Pergamon, and it states that the human body is composed of four fluids: blood, yellow bile, black bile, and phlegm. In a healthy person, these four humors are in balance, or *eucrasia*. In the opposite state, *dyscrasia*, the balance of the four humors is disturbed, causing sickness. This should be treated with a medicine designed to restore equilibrium. When diagnosing which of the four humors is out of balance, the temperament, personality, and other characteristics of the patient are also taken into account.

What Are Herbs?

Herbs are an extremely heterogeneous group of plants that include shrubs and woody plants as well as perennials, bulbs, and annuals. In medieval times, herbs were grown chiefly for medicinal purposes, with the emphasis on their curative properties—hence the common scientific suffix "officinalis." Monks showed great scientific rigor in this respect, painstakingly categorizing and labeling the plants. It is almost exclusively thanks to Hildegard of Bingen and her writings that this knowledge has been preserved. The monks planted their herbs separately in rectangular beds—a tradition that still survives to this day. Most herbs are ideal for this, being tidy, low-growing plants that look particularly attractive in a bed. With the ornamental gardens of the Early Modern period, herbs

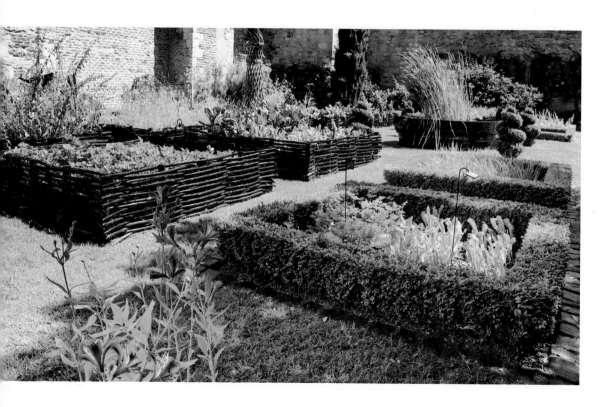

began to be planted purely for decorative purposes, in symmetrical patterns and usually in a terraced arrangement, until the focus returned to their culinary qualities and—following the rediscovery of Hildegard's writings—their healing qualities.

Medieval Medicine

Virtually all medicines of the medieval period were based on natural plant substances. Hildegard of Bingen took an almost scientific approach to these substances by the standards of the time, studying some two hundred different plants for their pharmacological efficacy. Some of these plants are still known to us as medicinal plants today, their potency having since been confirmed by the latest scientific methods. In other cases, however, we cannot know which plants Hildegard was referring to, since they are no longer known by the same names.

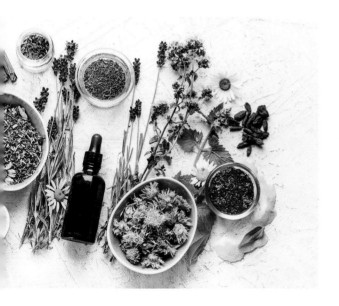

The Correct Use of Herbs

Hildegard of Bingen was particularly cautious with respect to high-potency herbs. She worked on the basis that if herbs were carelessly or incorrectly handled, their undisputed healing powers, which derive largely from their essential oils, could just as easily have the opposite effect and thus do more harm than good. For this reason, she stresses that medicinal herbs should be used to treat ailments only in the correct dosage and for a specific, limited period. Only then can certain herbs help combat certain diseases. Many of the herbs Hildegard describes are still used in herbal medicine today. Others have failed to prove effective by modern standards, and yet others have turned out to be even more effective than Hildegard described. This is due to the frame of reference she used for classification purposes: each of the herbs known at that time was assigned a temperature from warm to cold and a level of moisture from damp to dry. Any herb that could not be clearly assigned to these categories was therefore considered by Hildegard as useless or even harmful. However, this didn't stop the greatest medical practitioner of the Middle Ages from acting at all times according to her motto: "There is a herb for every ailment." With this in mind, she kept an array of herbs for treating all kinds of complaints in her herbal apothecary. And smaller quantities of herbs feature in nearly all of Hildegard's culinary recipes too—not just for seasoning but also for their capacity to ward off various diseases.

Healing Herbs for Every Ailment

In Hildegardian medicine, herbs are used not just for coughs and colds and stomach upsets but for all manner of pains and even inflammatory diseases. Stomach ailments are treated with parsley, stinging nettles, laurel, and mugwort; indigestion is combated with mugwort, basil, and licorice. Calendula and cumin help prevent flatulence. For patients suffering with a cold, Hildegard prescribes wild thyme, lovage, and licorice—particularly in case of coughs and hoarseness. Pellitory—a largely unknown herb nowadays—also brings relief from colds and inflammations of the respiratory tract. Infections of the lower respiratory tract are treated with lavender, cumin, and ground ivy; fever, with parsley and basil.

Earache is likewise relieved with ground ivy, while headaches call for laurel or wormwood. The latter is also good for toothache. Kidney problems are treated with elecampane. Lavender is said to be an effective liver medicine; nursing mothers should drink a milk-stimulating tea made from basil.

Skin problems are treated and soothed superficially with tinctures or poultices made from coltsfoot, elecampane, and wild thyme. For cases accompanied by suppuration or abscesses, Hildegard recommends verbena. Fresh skin wounds are treated with a tincture of yarrow—an herb that is still valued for its anti-inflammatory properties today. If the skin problems are due to insect bites, a tincture of plantain should be tried.

Saint-John's-wort is used in Hildegardian medicine—as elsewhere—to treat mild depression. Licorice, camphor, and lemon balm as well as hyssop can also help, however. For more serious cases, Hildegard recommends wormwood. Another common ailment in Hildegard's day was gout. This is treated with the healing herbs parsley, sage, mint, goutweed, and plantain. Hildegard even ventured to tackle paralysis, which she treated with thyme.

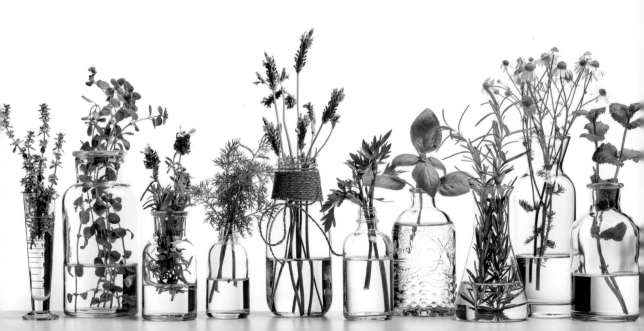

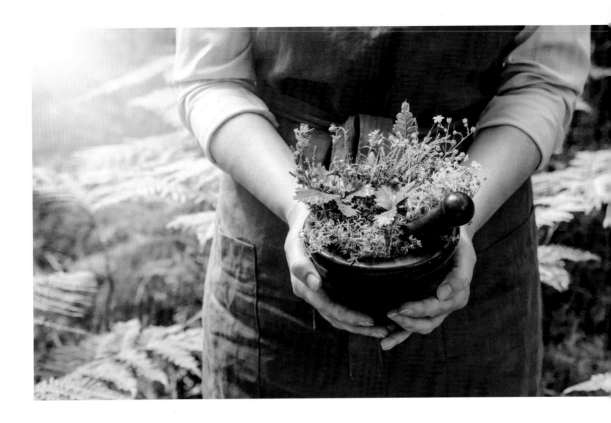

Getting the Dosage Right

It's not just about using the right herbs, however, but also using each one to optimal effect. In Hildegard's recipes, they are administered in the form of infusions, tinctures, compresses, and ointments or as a powder added to wine or water. Nor should we forget that Hildegard treated her patients without our modern knowledge of human anatomy or the precise composition of the herbs. Her nutritional therapy was based on observation, traditional lore, and experience. Many of her discoveries have stood up to subsequent scientific scrutiny. Some

Hildegard herbs are still used in modern herbalism—for example, in anti-inflammatory skin creams made with calendula, stomach-soothing teas with peppermint or chamomile, or cough-relieving teas with plantain, thyme, and sage. Even so, Hildegard's herbs should be used with caution, since some of their effects and side effects were not known to her then. Certain herbs such as tansy, rue, or hyssop should be avoided during pregnancy in particular.

Gardening with Hildegard of Bingen

Every garden should have a few of Hildegard's herbs. Most produce flowers that are every bit as pretty as those of purely ornamental plants. Their spicy, aromatic leaves lend the whole garden an intense, individual scent, depending on the chosen combination, and many of them have both culinary and health benefits when used in cooking. Hildegard herbs can be readily incorporated into any type of garden—there are no limits to the creative imagination. One of the most popular ways to arrange herbs is a terraced bed, which can be divided into several small sections by low hedges, narrow paths, or stone arrangements for a highly attractive visual effect. These separate small beds make it much easier to tend to and harvest the plants—all the more so because the different needs of each herb can be ideally accommodated. Herbs are also great for growing between other plants in a mixed border, however. Spherically or low-growing plants such as sage and chives work best in the foreground, while tall, stately plants such as lovage or fennel are good for providing structure. A hedge is an effective way of separating the entire herb garden from the rest of the garden. Thanks to their erect and rarely rampant growth, most herbs are perfect candidates for regularly arranged gardens, and their generally soft, subtle colors make them excellent companion plants for herbaceous borders. That said, they also do well amid the colorful confusion of natural garden concepts. Alternatively, if there is too little space in the garden for an herb bed, many Hildegard herbs can be planted in containers; most make excellent pot plants, and many also thrive in flower boxes.

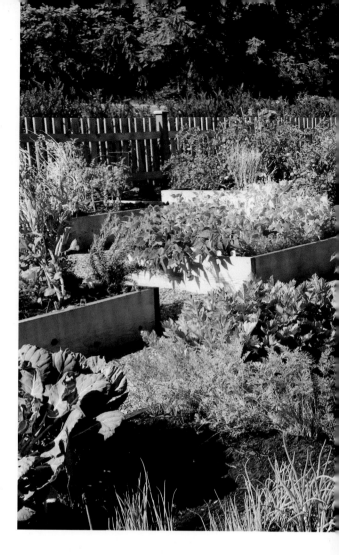

Positioning Your Herb Bed

The decision of where to position your herb bed within the garden is an important one. Bear in mind that many herbs originate from Mediterranean countries and are therefore used to a warm climate. These plants flourish best in the sunniest part of the garden. Others come from forest regions and prefer shady, damp locations. If the garden has heavy, water-retaining—and therefore cool—clay soil, it may be worth raising the beds to allow the water to drain more quickly from the root area. The hydraulic conductivity of the soil can be improved by digging in a mixture of gravel and sand.

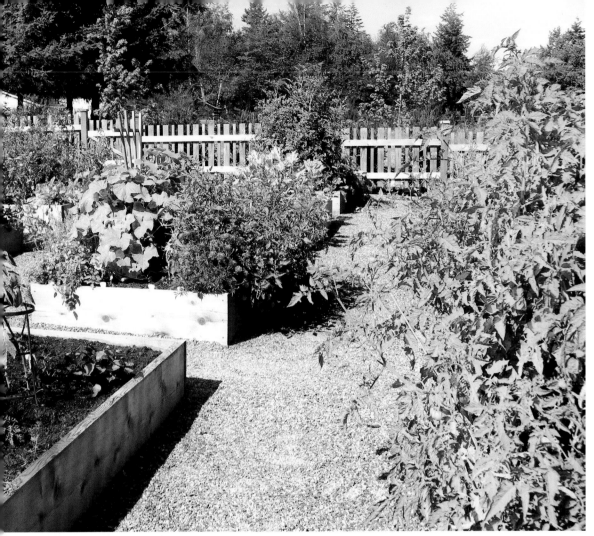

Through separate small garden beds, different needs can be met.

Many Hildegard herbs have a highly aromatic scent, which is intensified when the plants are brushed against or touched. For this reason, it is a good idea to plant a few larger, more robust herbs such as thyme, peppermint, or coriander next to the garden gate or alongside the paths. Creeping herbs such as wild thyme can be planted in the soil between stone slabs. For practicality, herbs that are used frequently in cooking can be planted in tubs, pots, or flower boxes close to the kitchen to save a trip around the garden each time herbs are needed.

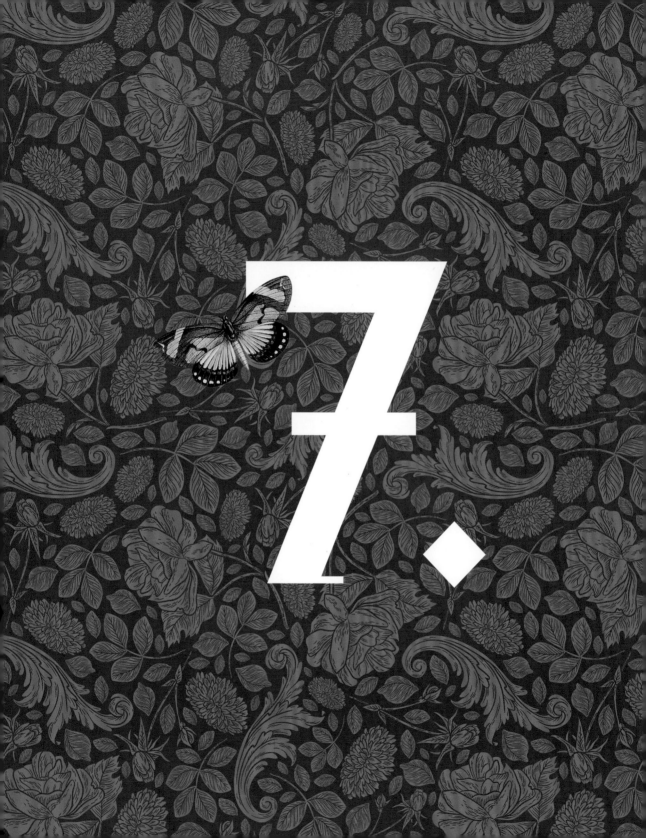

7.

HILDEGARD'S FAVORITE HERBS
FROM A TO Z

Basil *(Ocimum basilicum)*

A bushy annual growing up to 35 inches (90 centimeters [cm]) tall with thin, bright green pairs of leaves from 1 to 2 inches (2.5 to 5 cm) long, basil has small, white, tubular flowers. Its flowering season is from July to October. The leaves can be harvested continually as required, although the small, tender leaves have the most flavor. Basil is not frost resistant, and it should not be transferred to the herb bed until the risk of frost has passed and the weather has warmed. Plant the seedlings 10 inches (25 cm) apart in a sunny spot with sandy, nutrient-rich, moist soil and pinch out the shoot tips regularly. Hildegard recommends basil to protect against stroke and to treat feverish illnesses.

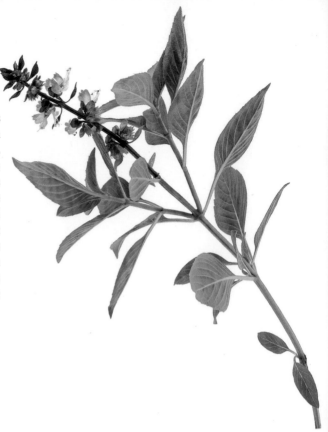

Bay Laurel *(Laurus nobilis)*

The laurel (or bay) tree originates from southern Europe. Its dark green leaves with their leathery sheen are narrowly ovate and up to 4 inches (10 cm) long. The tree flowers from March to May, producing clusters of small beige-colored flowers with yellow stamens. In cooler climates, laurel needs a sheltered, sunny location. The slow-growing shrub does not require any special care but should be protected in winter. Broken-off shoots and branches should be pruned at the end of the winter. The young leaves are traditionally used in dried form as a seasoning for sauces, marinades, soups, stews, and meat and fish dishes. In addition, Hildegard recommends making laurel wine by boiling the berries in wine. This is said to be particularly good for gastrointestinal complaints.

Brooklime *(Veronica beccabunga)*

A simple bog plant with hairless, fleshy leaves, this herbaceous perennial grows to a height of 8–24 inches (20–60 cm) and flowers from May onward. In the wild, brooklime—also known as horse cress—grows in boggy areas, near springs, along streams and rivers, and in ditches. The leaves can be used all year round. They are blanched briefly and seasoned with salt and garlic. Hildegard recommends brooklime for treating bleeding hemorrhoids.

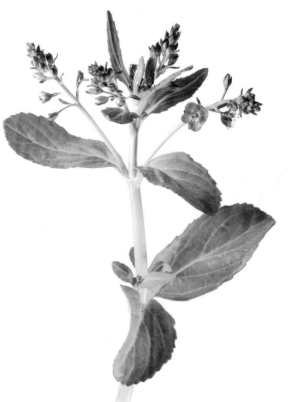

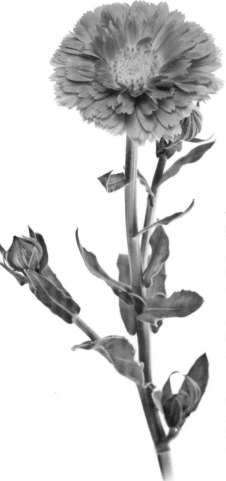

Calendula *(Calendula officinalis)*

A member of the daisy family, calendula or pot marigold is an annual plant growing to a maximum height of 28 inches (70 cm). It has an erect stem that branches only toward the top of the plant. The large, stalkless, obovate leaves are positioned alternately on the stem. Flowering begins in June and lasts into October. Each flower head contains around fifty individual disc florets, which are surrounded by yolk-yellow to orange-yellow ray florets.

Calendula is thought to originate from the Mediterranean, but it has been cultivated in central Europe since medieval times. It has also spread from gardens into the wild in some places. It is an easy plant to grow in the garden, being happy in most soils, but it should not be overfed, since this impairs flowering.

In natural medicine, the dried flower heads are used whole or crushed, along with the dried ray florets. These are then processed into teas, extracts, tinctures, and ointments. Calendula is used externally for wounds, bruises, inflammation, and rashes and internally for stomach and intestinal ulcers and menstrual problems. In addition, Hildegard recommends taking it internally to detoxify the body, particularly after food poisoning, and externally for improved skin health.

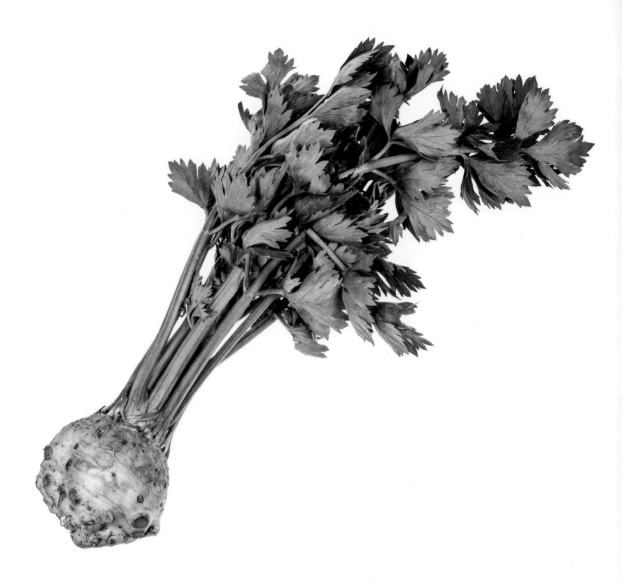

Celery/Celeriac *(Apium graveolens)*

Celery is a member of the *Umbelliferae* family, growing up to 3.3 feet (1 m) tall. It has been used for many centuries as a vegetable, condiment, and medicinal plant. There are three cultivars of the celery plant: celeriac, stalk celery, and leaf celery. The plant was already much prized by Hildegard: "Celery is a very juicy plant. It is not suitable for eating raw, but cooked celery is beneficial to human health." This assessment is backed up by modern research, which shows that celeriac in particular is rich in minerals and essential oils. Hildegard recommends the use of celery seeds for rheumatic pain. In addition, celery helps rid the body of excess fluid and acts as a diuretic. The closely related stalk celery can also be used, but it should always be steamed first.

Chervil *(Anthriscus cerefolium)*

This annual herb grows to a height of up to 24 inches (60 cm) and has light green feathery leaves, which can develop a pinkish-red tint when the seeds ripen. Chervil produces umbels of small white flowers throughout the summer. It prefers moist, nutrient-rich soil and semishade. The seeds are sown under glass in April, and the seedlings are planted outside 8 inches (20 cm) apart from late May onward. They should not be transplanted again. The first leaves can be harvested six weeks after germination and added in dried form to a variety of dishes. Hildegard is less interested in chervil's culinary uses than in its healing properties, however. For internal use, she advises mixing it with wine, to help heal "open wounds of the intestines." Otherwise, she recommends it for external use only, in order to treat skin diseases and ulcers.

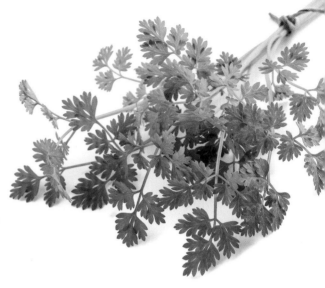

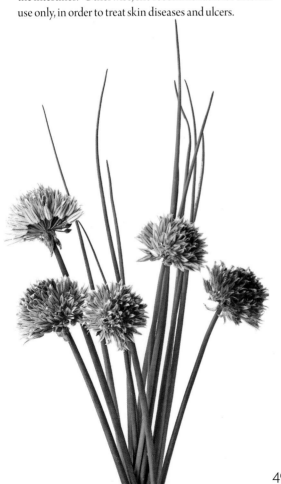

Chives *(Allium schoenoprasum)*

A bulbous plant with hollow, grasslike leaves up to 12 inches (30 cm) long, chives are sown under glass at the beginning of April and planted out in early summer. Regular cutting prevents the flowers from forming; otherwise, pretty pink inflorescences are produced in summer. The plant prefers sunny locations with chalky soils. Yellowing leaves mean that the lime content is too low. Chives also do well as a pot plant. The finely chopped leaves have a sharp, aromatic taste and are used in salads, in soups, and as a garnish on spreads. Hildegard recommends cooked chives for reviving the spirits and banishing melancholy.

Cinnamon *(Cinnamomum verum)*

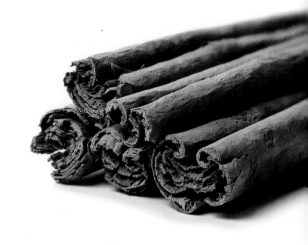

This spice is produced from the dried inner bark of the cinnamon tree. Originally exclusive to Sri Lanka, formerly known as Ceylon, the tree is now found in large areas of Southeast Asia and Central America. The bundled and fermented bark is dried in the sun, causing it to curl up into the familiar cinnamon sticks. Cinnamon is a very intense spice that lends itself particularly well to compotes, desserts, baked goods, and punches. Its medicinal value was discovered 2,500 years ago by the Greek physician Hippocrates. The essential oil contained in the tree bark has an anti-inflammatory, warming effect and serves to stimulate circulation and digestion. For general fortification and particularly in cases of gout, Hildegard recommends hot wine with cinnamon—essentially mulled wine.

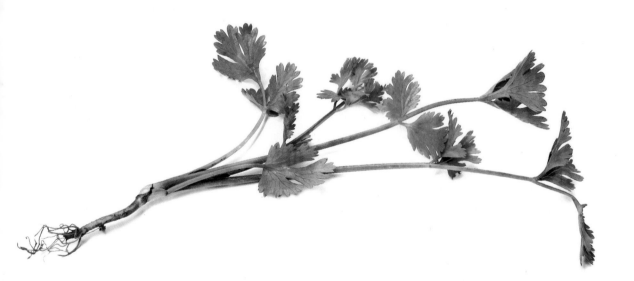

Coriander *(Coreandrum sativum)*

This annual herb grows to a height of up to 24 inches (60 cm). It has broad, shiny leaves at the base of the plant and thin, threadlike ones toward the top. Umbels of small pink flowers appear in high summer. The leaves are harvested as needed up to the flowering season, and they are used in dried form to flavor a variety of meat dishes. The seed, which is used to flavor marinades and desserts, has an unpleasant smell when unripe, and a slight note of aniseed when ripe. In Hildegardian medicine, coriander serves to help detoxify the body.

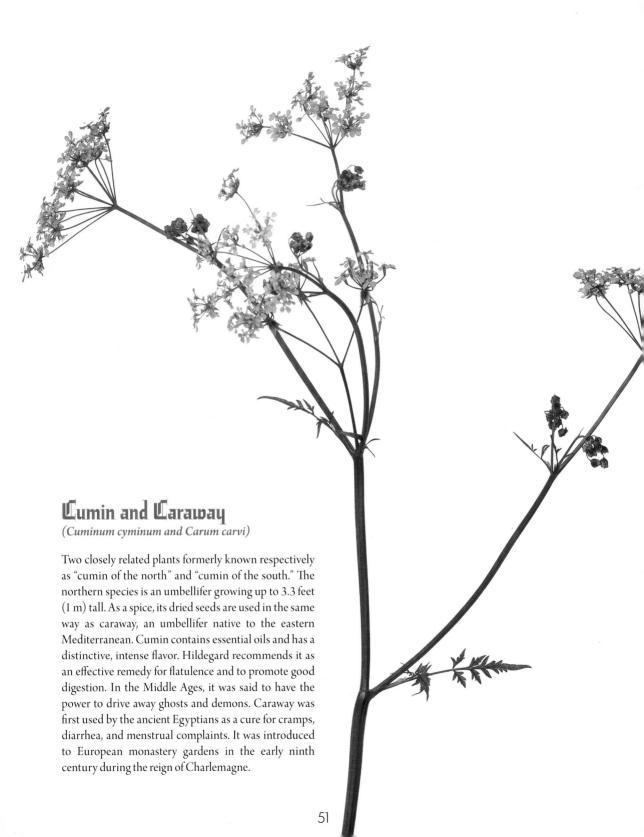

Cumin and Caraway
(Cuminum cyminum and Carum carvi)

Two closely related plants formerly known respectively as "cumin of the north" and "cumin of the south." The northern species is an umbellifer growing up to 3.3 feet (1 m) tall. As a spice, its dried seeds are used in the same way as caraway, an umbellifer native to the eastern Mediterranean. Cumin contains essential oils and has a distinctive, intense flavor. Hildegard recommends it as an effective remedy for flatulence and to promote good digestion. In the Middle Ages, it was said to have the power to drive away ghosts and demons. Caraway was first used by the ancient Egyptians as a cure for cramps, diarrhea, and menstrual complaints. It was introduced to European monastery gardens in the early ninth century during the reign of Charlemagne.

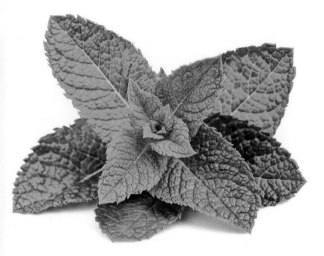

Curly Mint *(Mentha crispa)*

Named for its frilled leaves, this herbaceous perennial reaches a height of up to 24 inches (60 cm). It grows in well-watered soil in woodland margins and scrubland. In the garden, it needs semishade and nutrient-rich, moist soil. The leaves are gathered before the beginning of the flowering season in August, and they are added, finely chopped, to meat, game, and fish dishes as well as sauces, soups, and stews. Hildegard recommends curly mint for stomach problems and also for digestive complaints.

Dill *(Anethum graveolens)*

Approximately 3 feet (1 m) tall, this annual has highly feathered leaves. The flowers are small and yellowish in color and borne on flat, umbel-like clusters, which appear from June to August. Dill is a low-maintenance, self-seeding plant that thrives in sunny locations, even in meager, dry soils. It grows particularly fast during hot summers and should be protected from strong winds. Dill leaves can be harvested as soon as the plant is 10–12 inches (25–30 cm) tall. For pickling cucumber, it needs to be picked when in flower and in dry conditions. Hildegard warns against consuming the herb raw and recommends sauces with cooked dill to help alleviate rheumatism.

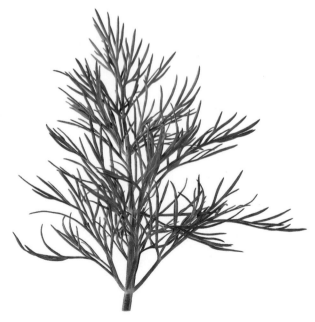

Dittany *(Dictamnus albus)*

This herbaceous perennial belongs to the rue family and is a close relative of the citrus family. It grows to a height of up to 3.3 feet (1 m) and has odd-pinnate leaves. The flowers grow up to 2 inches (5 cm) long, are pink in color, and appear from May to June. They are borne on long, eye-catching inflorescences and have an intense citrus scent. Dittany needs plenty of sun and warmth. In the garden, it needs a prime, well-sheltered location. According to Hildegard, it can be used in dried, powdered form to normalize high blood lipid levels and prevent arteriosclerosis.

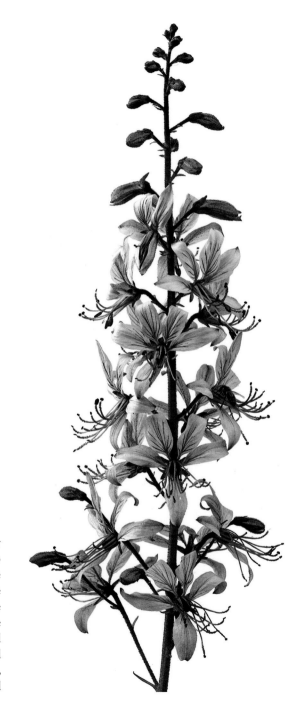

Galangal *(Alpinia officinarum)*

Galangal originates from southern China, Indonesia, and India and is a member of the ginger family. The root, being the useful part of the plant, is thought to have reached Europe in the early Middle Ages. It contains pungent aromatic compounds and potent essential oils and can help relieve cramps, improve digestion, and alleviate the effects of stress. It also has pain-relieving properties. It is perhaps mostly valued, however, for its highly beneficial effect on the heart. It is used for heart problems including angina and helps prevent heart attacks. Also available in concentrated tablet form, it is said to be just as effective in this respect as conventional nitroglycerin preparations but without their unpleasant side effects. In addition, galangal can relieve cramps in the digestive tract, ease menstrual problems in women, and reduce general weakness. Hildegard recommends adding one to three pinches of galangal powder to food, and it also makes for a spicy seasoning. For fever and pain, she recommends galangal wine. Last but not least, galangal is one of the components of Hildegard's Ginger Mix Powder.

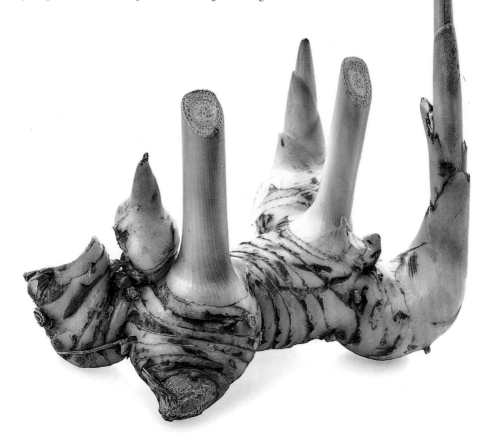

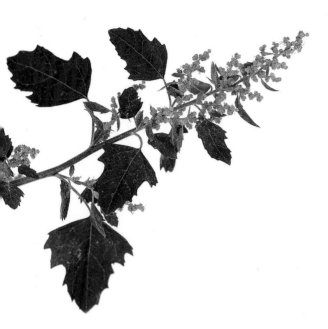

Garden Orach (*Atriplex hortensis*)

Cultivated in gardens for centuries as "French spinach," garden orach, which grows to a height of up to 3.3 feet (1 m), has since been almost entirely displaced and is now regarded at best as a weed. A low-maintenance annual plant, it has mealy-looking, triangular to heart-shaped leaves and thrives in almost any soil. The leaves are harvested and eaten raw or in salads. In Hildegardian medicine, they are used to normalize digestion and fortify the immune system.

Garlic (*Allium sativum*)

Familiar bulb with broad, grasslike leaves borne on a thick flowering stem up to 20 inches (50 cm) tall. The bulb consists of several cloves covered in a whitish skin. Garlic flowers from July to August, producing pinkish-white flower heads. The bulbs are planted in late summer and fall at a depth of 2–4 inches (5–10 cm) in nutrient-rich soil, which should be well fertilized once a year. The seedlings are then moved to a cold frame in the spring and must be watered frequently during dry periods. The plants should be divided every three to four years and transplanted. The ripe bulbs are dug up in late summer. Hildegard warns against cooked garlic and recommends using it raw in order to improve vitality, lower blood pressure, and help prevent arteriosclerosis.

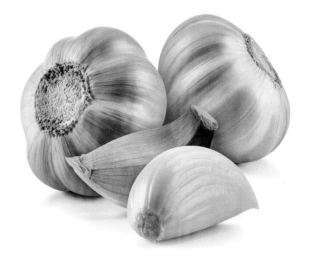

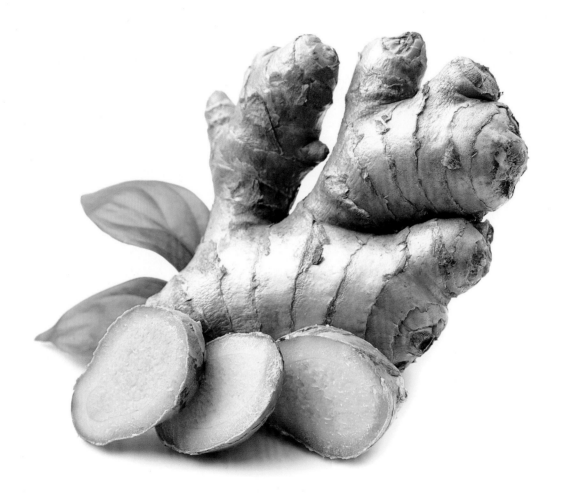

Ginger *(Zingiber officinale)*

Ginger is an herbaceous perennial from Southeast Asia. It has a reed-like structure and is widely cultivated from India through China to Japan as well as Australia, South America, and West Africa. The usable part of the plant is the rhizome, a kind of underground central organ that is commonly known as the root. Ginger root was known to Mediterranean countries from antiquity, and it came to central Europe via the Alps in the early ninth century. It has mild psychoactive properties and is said to suppress the rational side of the human psyche while boosting the emotional side. For this reason, Hildegard recommends using it only in small quantities. Ginger's healing power lies in its ability to fortify people suffering from weakness. In Hildegard's Ginger Mix Powder, it is mixed with galangal and zedoary and helps relieve eye problems, constipation, and colic. Today, it is also known for its expectorant effect on coughs and colds and its anti-inflammatory and pain relief effects on arthrosis and rheumatism. New varieties of ginger have recently been introduced that are able to thrive in colder climates, although these have not yet become established in private gardens.

Greater Burnet-Saxifrage
(Pimpinella major)

This herbaceous perennial grows up to 3.3 feet (1 m) tall with ridged stems and pinnate leaves. The stem grows out of rosette of basal leaves. The flowers appear in June and last into September. The tiny white single flowers are clustered in umbel-like inflorescences. In the garden, the plant needs a loamy, nutrient-rich soil and a sunny location. Hildegard recommends using the rootstock and roots, which are rich in essential oils. They are used as a vegetable or salad green, as well as in dried and powdered form as a tea or gargling solution. Their main application is for throat and bronchial infections.

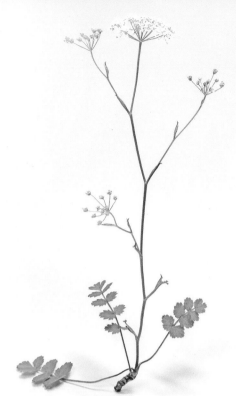

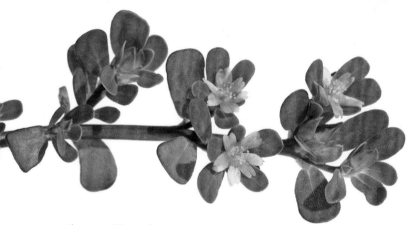

Green Purslane *(Portulaca oleracea)*

Annual plant growing up to 24 inches (60 cm) tall with fleshy, sessile ovate leaves. Green purslane is of Asian origin, but it has since spread throughout the world. In the garden, it prefers light, warm, and sandy soils in sheltered, sunny locations. The seeds are sown directly outdoors once the risk of frost has passed, and the plants must be watered regularly. The leaves are harvested before the onset of the flowering season in August. They are used either as a salad vegetable or chopped up as a condiment in salads, soups, sauces, and broths. The leaves should not be added too early during cooking, because they can lose much of their flavor. Although Hildegard considered purslane, which she referred to as *Burtel*, to have no nutritional or medicinal benefits, it was later discovered to help relieve digestive complaints.

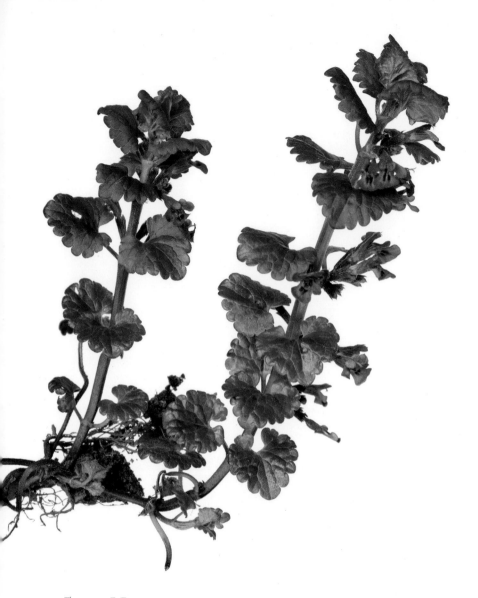

Ground Ivy *(Glechoma hederacea)*

Known in medieval times as "Old Lady's Vine," ground ivy grows to a height of just 12 inches (30 cm). Commonly found in the wild, it has oppositely arranged, scalloped, kidney-shaped leaves, sometimes with a reddish or brownish tint. It grows along woodland margins, waysides, and riverbanks. In the garden, ground ivy needs semishade and nutrient-rich soil. Its purple flowers appear in the leaf axils as early as March. It remains in flower until May and is harvested during this time. It can be added to food in very small quantities and can also be used as a bath additive. Both applications are recommended for persistent weakness, particularly in the elderly. In addition, Hildegard recommends an infusion of ground ivy for lung and throat conditions as well as ear infections, due to the plant's anti-inflammatory and expectorant properties. It is also used to alleviate toothache and relieve tinnitus, dizziness, and spring fever.

Horseradish *(Armoracia rusticana)*

Horseradish is a highly resilient cruciferous plant that can grow up to 6.5 feet (2 m) tall. It is a perennial plant whose overwintering organ takes the form of a long, taproot-like rhizome. This highly aromatic root is used as a vegetable, condiment, and medicinal herb. Hildegard recommends it for seasonal use only, and the season is limited to the early spring, when the root is softer and less woody than at other times of the year. As Hildegard notes, "In March, when all herbs are in bud, the horseradish also softens, but only for a short time. Then it is good for the healthy and strong because it fortifies their vital energy. When it grows hard and tough, however, it is dangerous to eat, having lost all its healing power."

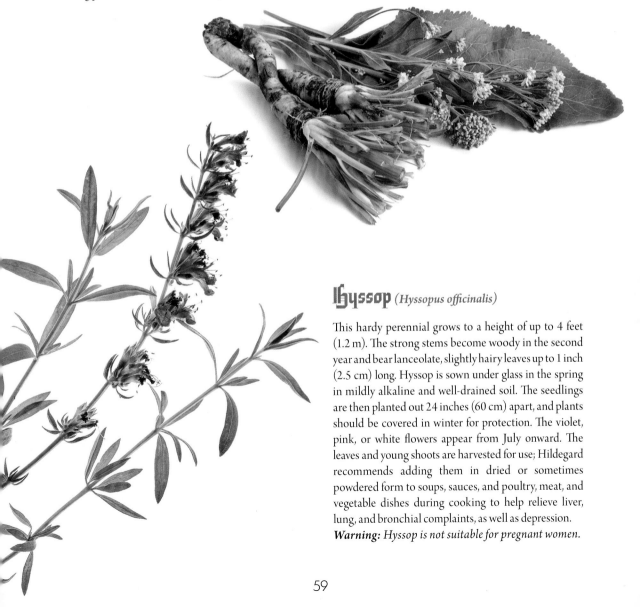

Hyssop *(Hyssopus officinalis)*

This hardy perennial grows to a height of up to 4 feet (1.2 m). The strong stems become woody in the second year and bear lanceolate, slightly hairy leaves up to 1 inch (2.5 cm) long. Hyssop is sown under glass in the spring in mildly alkaline and well-drained soil. The seedlings are then planted out 24 inches (60 cm) apart, and plants should be covered in winter for protection. The violet, pink, or white flowers appear from July onward. The leaves and young shoots are harvested for use; Hildegard recommends adding them in dried or sometimes powdered form to soups, sauces, and poultry, meat, and vegetable dishes during cooking to help relieve liver, lung, and bronchial complaints, as well as depression.
Warning: Hyssop is not suitable for pregnant women.

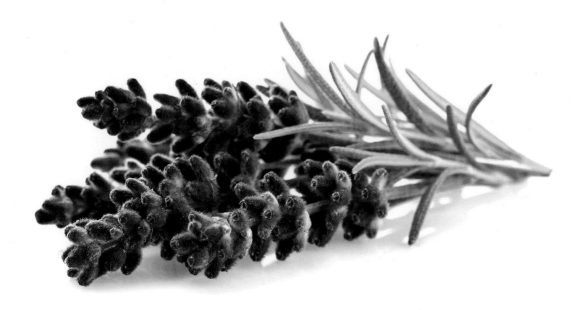

Lavender (*Lavandula augustifolia*)

Lavender originates from the Mediterranean coast, where it grows wild on dry, rocky slopes. Nowadays it is also cultivated there on a large scale. It was introduced to central Europe via the Alps by Benedictine monks; in that area, the plant now grows almost exclusively in gardens, escaping only very rarely into the wild. This hardy perennial is a bushy shrub growing up to 35 inches (90 cm) tall. The woody, multibranched shoots have oppositely arranged, linear, gray-green leaves. During the flowering season, the intensely aromatic blue-violet flowers appear on spikes that are 2 inches (5 cm) long.

To thrive in the garden, lavender needs as much sun as possible and a dry, slightly chalky soil. The flowering season lasts from July to November. Hildegard recommends harvesting the leaves and shoot tips before its onset; the flower itself should be harvested until the end of August. Although winter hardy, plants grown in pots or containers should be brought indoors or covered during the cold season to protect them from freezing temperatures, because once the roots become frost-damaged, the plant grows sickly and susceptible to a variety of diseases and pests.

Lavender flowers have a long history as a moth repellent, and lavender extract is also thought to deter head lice. The dried flowers and leaves are used to flavor marinades, meat, fish, and vegetable dishes. Lavender tea is recommended by Hildegard for liver and lung complaints, and the plant also features in Hildegard's natural cosmetics. Please note, however, that it can be a major skin irritant if used in very high concentrations (for example, as an oil).

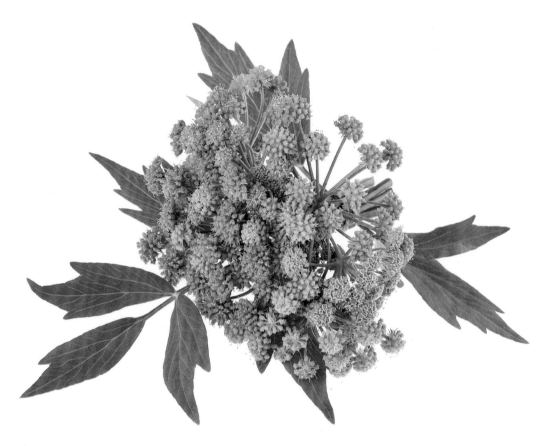

Lovage *(Levisticum officinale)*

This hardy perennial can grow to a height of 6.5 feet (2 m). The tripartite leaves can be up to 24 inches (60 cm) long and are borne on erect stems. From June to August, lovage produces a mass of small yellow flowers arranged in umbel-like inflorescences. It was probably brought to Europe from the Persian region via the Mediterranean during Hildegard's lifetime and introduced from there to central Europe, where it quickly became established in monastery gardens.

The plants should be sown in small seedling trays and not planted out until six weeks later. Lovage is fairly low maintenance and also thrives in semishade, though it prefers a sunny location. The plants need occasional feeding and should be covered during sharp frosts. All parts of the plant may be used. The tender young leaflets are harvested throughout the summer, until the flowers or roots appear in the fall. The seeds are harvested in the fall, once ripened.

Lovage is much less popular nowadays than in past centuries, when it was used as a universal cooking ingredient. In medieval times, the plant was considered an aphrodisiac due to its strong scent and was used by women to attract men. On the culinary front, Hildegard recommends it for virtually all aromatic dishes. For medicinal purposes, she used the leaves in the form of an herb tea to treat abdominal and menstrual problems, as well as coughs, digestive disorders, and headaches.

Warning: *Lovage should not be used by pregnant women due to its stimulating effect on the uterus.*

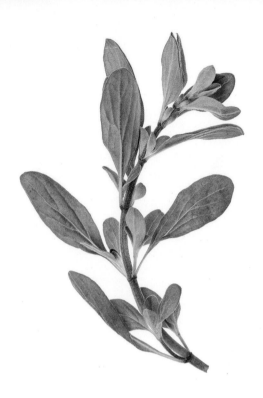

Marjoram *(Origanum majorana)*

This compact, branched subshrub with woody stems grows to a height of up to approximately 20 inches (50 cm). The oppositely arranged leaves are gray green, soft, ovate, and between 2 and 8 inches (6 and 20 cm) long. Marjoram produces inconspicuous pink or white flowers from June to September. It is mildly cold sensitive, and it should be sown under glass initially and not planted out until mid- to late May. The seedlings should be planted 8 inches (20 cm) apart in nutrient-rich soil in a sunny, sheltered location. The soil must be kept well watered. The best times of day for harvesting are morning and late afternoon, because this is when the leaves have the highest oil content. The fresh or dried leaves are added to meat, vegetable, or fish dishes.

Masterwort *(Peucedanum ostruthium)*

Masterwort is an umbellifer from the Alpine region that grows to a height of up to 3.3 feet (1 m). It originally occurred exclusively at altitudes above 4,600 feet (1,400 m) but has also been cultivated as a medicinal plant since the Middle Ages. The root is used in herbal liqueurs and made into powders, extracts, and ointments. Hildegard recommends masterwort crushed in wine for fever and in combination with ginger for digestive complaints of all kinds. In the garden, the plant, which produces decorative flowers in July and August, needs plenty of sun; a dry, not-too-nutrient-rich soil; and lots of space, since it spreads rapidly via underground runners.

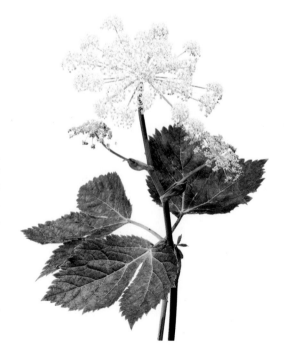

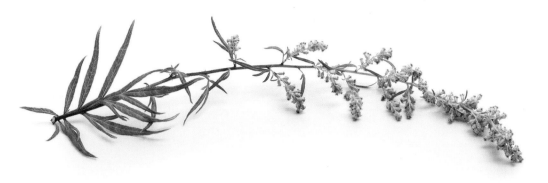

Mugwort *(Artemisia vulgaris)*

Growing up to 8 feet (2.5 m) tall, this perennial has broad, hairless leaves that have a fluffy white underside and yellowish to red-brown flowers with downy hairs. Its flowering season runs from July to September. Mugwort is a low-maintenance plant, but it grows best in sunny conditions. The leaves of the plant are harvested and stored in dried form in very small quantities. The flowers should not be used due to their extreme bitterness. Mugwort aids the digestion of fats and therefore tends to be used with particularly fatty foods such as roast goose or duck. It is also recommended by Hildegard for treating chronic digestive problems.

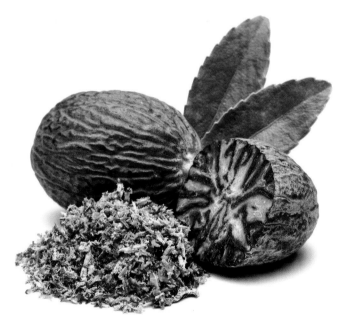

Nutmeg *(Myristica fragrans)*

Nutmeg is the seed of the nutmeg tree and grows like a stone inside a peach-like fruit. The nutmeg tree lives for a hundred years, reaches a height of 49 feet (15 m), and originates from the Maluku Islands ("Spice Islands"). Today, it is cultivated in large parts of the Southeast Asian archipelago and in Brazil. Nutmeg has even been found in the graves of ancient Egyptian mummies. Grated nutmeg is a spice that is used very sparingly and lends a characteristic warmth to a variety of dishes. According to Hildegard, its main medicinal uses are for depression, poisoning, weakness, and digestive complaints. It is psychoactive if consumed to excess and can induce mild intoxication with hallucinations. Extreme overdosing can lead to severe poisoning and even death.

Onion (*Allium cepa*)

Onions are almost as good for you as their close relative garlic. They contain sulfur compounds with antibiotic properties and digestion-friendly essential oils, and they serve to lower blood pressure as well as to reduce blood fat and cholesterol levels. Onions also contain an array of vitamins and minerals. Finally, they stimulate the appetite, act as a diuretic, loosen bronchial mucous, and lower high temperatures due to coughs and colds. Externally, they are traditionally used in "onion packs" to treat middle-ear infections. According to Hildegard, all the above remedies require the onions to be cooked; she maintains that "in its raw state, the onion is as harmful and toxic as a weed."

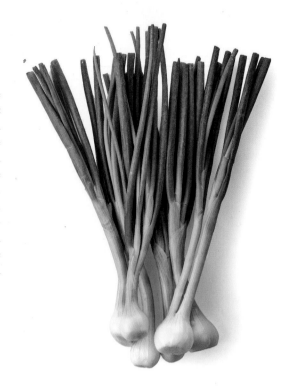

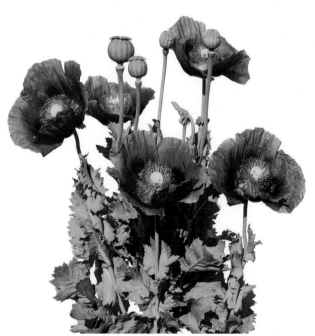

Opium Poppy (*Papaver somniferum*)

A well-known medicinal and aromatic plant, this biennial is now cultivated almost exclusively as an ornamental plant in the West. The use of the opium poppy is somewhat problematic due to the fact that all parts of the plant except the seeds contain extremely dangerous substances including opium, codeine, and heroin. The nontoxic seeds, on the other hand, are recommended by Hildegard when fully ripened for itching and insomnia.
Warning: Due to the risk of poisoning and in conformity with drug laws, only the seeds of the opium poppy should be used and no other part of the plant.

Parsley *(Petroselinum sp.)*

This hardy annual or biennial plant grows up to 12 inches (30 cm) tall and has flat or curly compound leaves. Parsley is sown in April in deep, highly nutrient-rich soil and prefers sun or semishade. The seeds germinate after approximately six weeks, and the seedlings are thinned out to 12 inches (30 cm) apart. Parsley should always be kept well watered. The leaves and stems can be picked as needed throughout the summer but become bitter once the plant is in flower. Raw parsley provides a subtle flavoring for almost any savory dish, but it should not be added during cooking since it soon loses its piquancy. Flat-leaf parsley has a stronger flavor than the curly variety. Parsley root, too, is highly aromatic. Parsley is recommended by Hildegard for fortifying the cardiovascular system and in case of fever. A good way to take it is in the form of parsley and honey wine, made by boiling the herb in wine with honey.

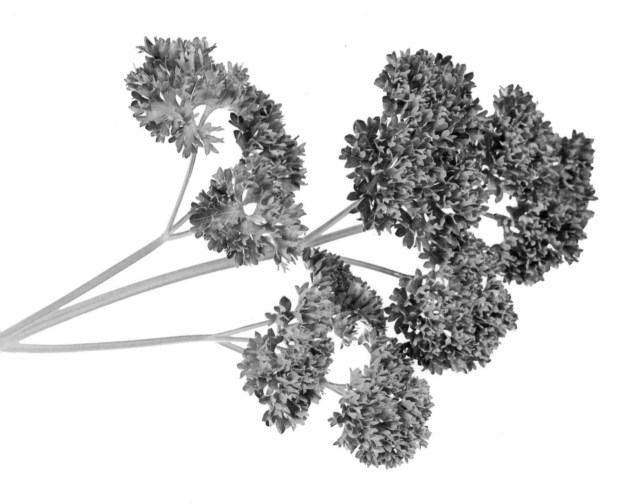

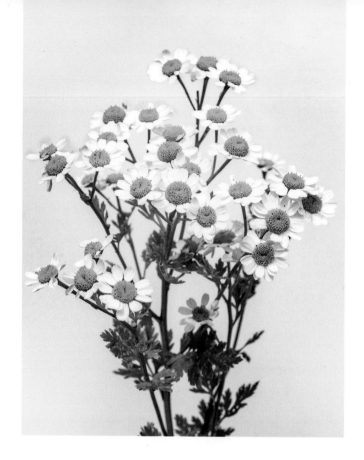

Pellitory *(Anacyclus officinarum/pyrethrum)*

Without a doubt, pellitory, or *Bertram* in German, is the most mysterious plant in the Hildegardian pharmacopeia. Why? Because this herb, prescribed by Hildegard for all manner of ailments, no longer exists. Pellitory is sometimes assumed to have been another name for tarragon, but this does not appear to be the case. In fact, German pellitory (*A. officinarum*) existed until the end of the nineteenth century, being cultivated in the area around Magdeburg for the medicinal properties of its root. In the 1890s, it appears to have died out there, and the plant has since disappeared. From the outside, this member of the daisy family closely resembles chamomile, and it was perhaps because of this confusion that its disappearance initially went unnoticed. Hildegard's German pellitory was probably a cultivar of perennial pellitory (*A. pyrethrum*), which occurs in western Mediterranean countries and is still grown today as a medicinal plant in Spain and Morocco. Hildegard recommended pellitory for the general fortification of body and mind and specifically for digestive complaints, coughs and colds, and eye problems. The ground root of modern pellitory is a pungent spice that is also occasionally used in herb liqueurs. In addition to the alkaloid pyrethrin, pellitory root contains essential oils and the polysaccharide insulin. Pellitory is used to improve digestion, for anemia, and as a complementary treatment for diabetes. One to three pinches of powdered pellitory are added to soups, sauces, or grain dishes during cooking or sprinkled on top before serving. It is also good for scattering over loaves of bread. In powdered form, pellitory can be stored for long periods. In the garden, this low-growing, creeping, and extremely robust plant with its strong taproot fares best in a dry and sunny rock garden.

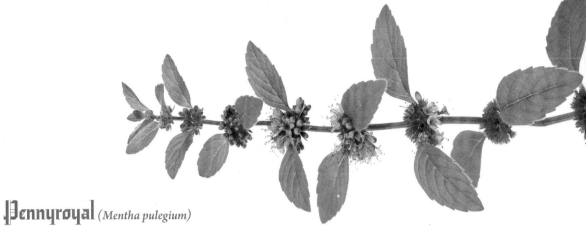

Pennyroyal *(Mentha pulegium)*

This low-growing herbaceous perennial grows to approximately 6–16 inches (15–40 cm). Clusters of flowers appear in the upper third of the stem and shoots and in the leaf axils from July. In the garden, pennyroyal needs sun or semishade and must be kept well watered. Its leaves and shoot tips are harvested before the onset of the flowering season and added in dried form to vegetable and meat dishes, sauces, and savory marinades. It is recommended by Hildegard particularly for gastrointestinal and gallbladder complaints. ***Warning:*** *Caution should be taken with pennyroyal, and it should be avoided by those who are pregnant. Pennyroyal oil is toxic and should not be ingested.*

Peppermint *(Mentha piperita)*

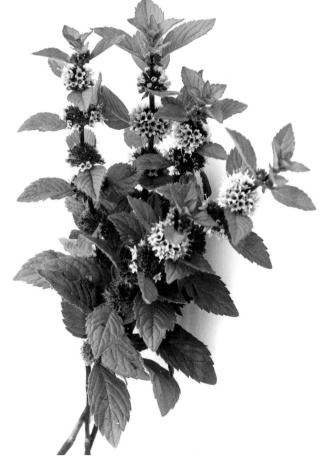

Hildegard cannot have been familiar with this herbaceous perennial, which grows to 30 inches (75 cm) tall, because it wasn't bred until the end of the seventeenth century, hundreds of years after her death, by crossing spearmint with water mint. She was, however, familiar with pennyroyal, which is similar to peppermint but has fallen out of favor due to its higher amounts of pulegone (a natural pesticide). Peppermint can serve as a substitute. Its dark green leaves are oppositely arranged, coarsely toothed, and hairy on both sides, and they can be up to 3 inches (8 cm) long. The seedlings are best obtained from a nursery and planted in spring in loamy soil at a depth of roughly 2 inches (5 cm) and a distance of 8–12 inches (20–30 cm) apart. Peppermint loves the sun and needs to be watered regularly. The plants should be replaced every three to four years to avoid fungal attacks. The flowers are bluish violet and appear from July onward. The leaves are harvested until shortly before the flowering season, preferably in the morning or late afternoon, when their essential oil content is highest. Peppermint is added to food, or it can be drunk as a tea, particularly in case of stomach upsets and feverish colds.

Rosemary *(Rosmarinus officinalis)*

This hardy evergreen shrub can grow up to 6.5 feet (2 m) tall and has resinous, needle-shaped leaves on woody stems. The blue to violet flowers appear in May and last until July. In May, when the risk of frost is past, cuttings are planted outdoors in moist soil at an interval of 20 inches (50 cm) apart. Rosemary needs as much sun as possible, and the soil should be kept moist but not wet. It can freeze in particularly hard winters and should be covered. It also does well as a pot plant, because it can then be moved to a suitable indoor spot during the colder months. The shoots are harvested and added in fresh, dried, or powdered form to any savory dish and to sauces, marinades, and pickles. Hildegard recommends rosemary for its expectorant effect on coughs and colds, as well as for digestive and menstrual complaints.

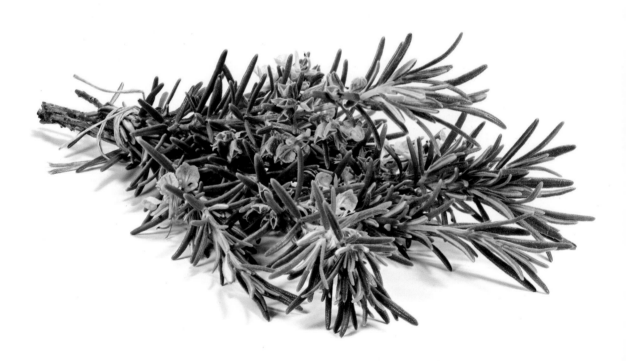

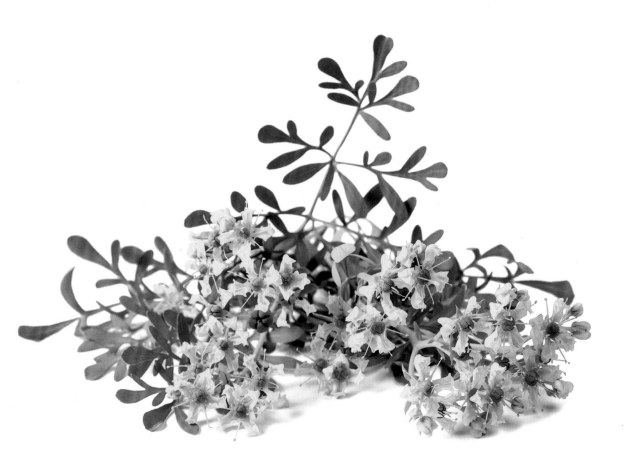

Rue *(Ruta graveolens)*

Rutaceous plant of southern European origin, close relative of the citrus family. This bushy perennial subshrub grows to a height of 3.3 feet (1 m). The fleshy leaves are strongly pinnate. Rue needs a sunny, sheltered location and a nutrient-rich, moist but not wet soil. The leaves contain a very high concentration of essential oils and should be used only in small doses, whether fresh or dried. They are added to meat, fish, and vegetable dishes and to salads, pickles, dairy products, and spreads. Hildegard recommends rue for cardiovascular complaints, digestive problems, stomach and gallbladder disorders, menstrual and menopausal problems, and mood swings.

Warning: Rue is not suitable for pregnant women.

Sage *(Salvia officinalis)*

This perennial plant originating from the Mediterranean region has thick stems turning woody at the base. The green-gray leaves are oblong-ovate with slightly crinkled edges, and they have a distinctive soft, bumpy surface. The seedlings should not be transferred from the nursery until the second half of May, when the risk of late overnight frosts is past, and should be planted approximately 16 inches (40 cm) apart. Sage prefers a warm, sunny location with a well-drained, calcareous, sandy soil. It needs very little watering. Regular pruning will encourage new growth. From June onward, it produces mauve to blue-violet flowers in terminal, spikelike inflorescences. The leaves are used fresh or dried, and they can be added to almost any hearty dish or used to make a tea. In the Hildegardian kitchen, sage is used to purify the bodily fluids, treat sore throats and stomach complaints, and protect against infection.

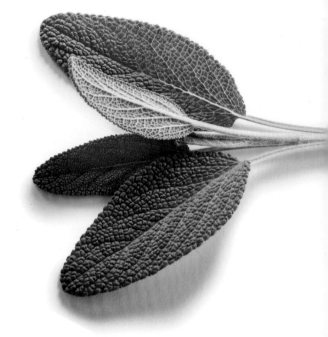

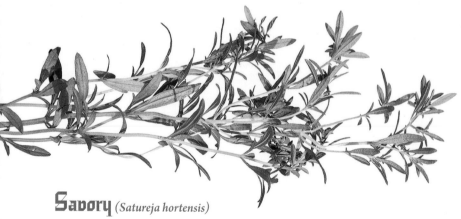

Savory *(Satureja hortensis)*

An aromatic, nonhardy annual with rounded leaves, savory grows to a height of approximately 18 inches (45 cm) and produces small pale lilac to white flowers in late summer. The flowering season lasts for several weeks. Savory is sown under glass and should not be planted outside until the risk of late overnight frosts is judged to be past. The seedlings are planted approximately 8 inches (20 cm) apart. Savory thrives in well-drained, nutrient-poor soil. The harvested leaves and shoots are recommended by Hildegard as a digestive aid that can be used to flavor meat dishes and especially pulses (the dried seeds of legume plants). In powdered form, savory can be added to cumin and sage powder mixed with honey to help prevent gout, rheumatism, and Parkinson's disease. It is also used to treat cardiovascular diseases and mood swings.

Spignel *(Meum athamanticum)*

This hardy perennial reaches a height of 8–20 inches (20–50 cm). The green stems are round and finely grooved, and the feathery leaves give off an intensive scent when rubbed. The thick rootstock is said to have been a delicacy for bears once upon a time (hence the German name *Bärwurz* or "bear wort"). Flowering in large colonies from May to July, spignel is confined to specific geographical regions, growing in the acidic, nutrient-poor meadows of some upland areas. In the garden, spignel needs a sunny location and a meager soil with a low lime content. The powdered root is used in savory spreads or as a soup seasoning to protect against feverish conditions, gout, and liver ailments (hepatitis). Hildegard's famous remedy made from powdered spignel, cooked pear puree, and honey is used for general detoxification of the body.

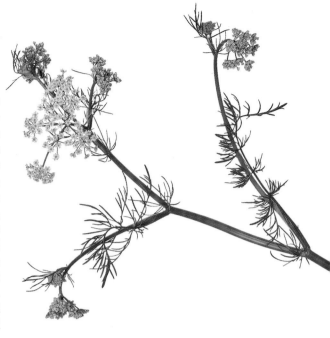

Stinging Nettle *(Urtica dioica)*

Roughly 24 inches (60 cm) tall, this annual has elongated, heart-shaped, dark green leaves, both sides of which are covered with a thick layer of stinging hairs. The tips of the hairs can penetrate the skin, thereby releasing the fluid contained in the stinging cells, which causes the familiar red, blistery rash. The plain, greenish flowers appear on catkin-like heads from June to September. Stinging nettles favor nutrient-rich soils in semishade. They are self-seeding and also spread via underground runners. Gloves should always be worn when harvesting the young shoots and leaves. These are gathered from March to June, before flowering, and should always be cooked before consuming. According to Hildegard, they can then be used either as a condiment or as a salad green or vegetable, and they are excellent for purifying the blood and treating stomach complaints.

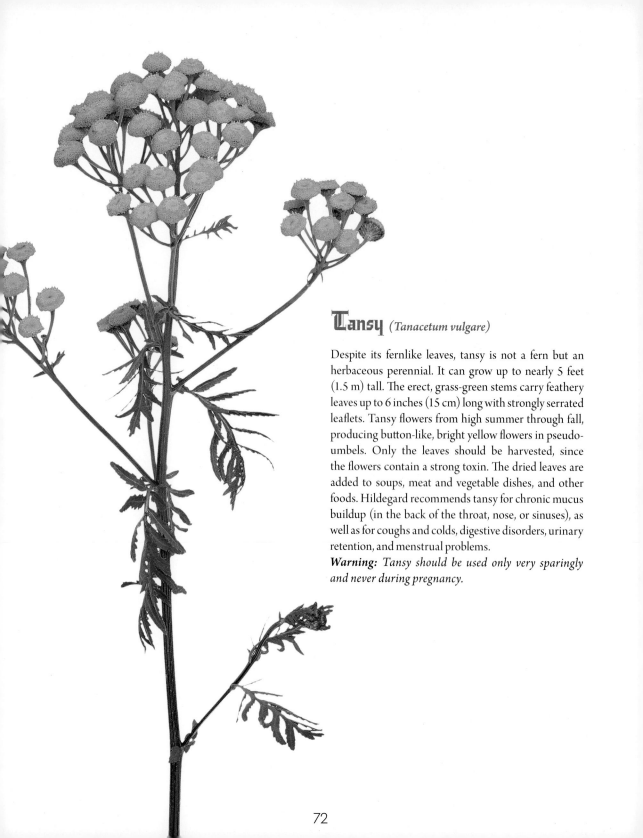

Tansy *(Tanacetum vulgare)*

Despite its fernlike leaves, tansy is not a fern but an herbaceous perennial. It can grow up to nearly 5 feet (1.5 m) tall. The erect, grass-green stems carry feathery leaves up to 6 inches (15 cm) long with strongly serrated leaflets. Tansy flowers from high summer through fall, producing button-like, bright yellow flowers in pseudo-umbels. Only the leaves should be harvested, since the flowers contain a strong toxin. The dried leaves are added to soups, meat and vegetable dishes, and other foods. Hildegard recommends tansy for chronic mucus buildup (in the back of the throat, nose, or sinuses), as well as for coughs and colds, digestive disorders, urinary retention, and menstrual problems.

Warning: Tansy should be used only very sparingly and never during pregnancy.

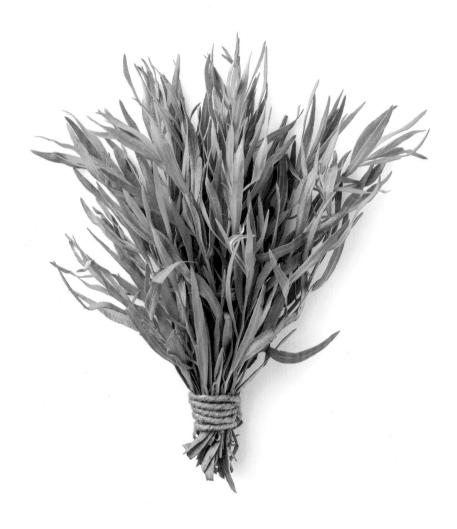

Tarragon *(Artemisia dracunculus)*

This perennial herb growing to a height of 5 feet (1.5 m) has erect, bushy, branched stems and pointed, dark green leaves. The inconspicuous greenish-yellow flowers appear in loose clusters from July onward. The seeds are sown under glass from April, in loose, damp, chalky, and humus-rich soil. The seedlings are planted outside 16 inches (40 cm) apart. Tarragon needs a sunny location sheltered from cold winds. The plants should be divided and transplanted after three to four years at the latest, since they will otherwise soon deteriorate. The leaves and young shoots are harvested and used in dried form as a highly delicate seasoning. Tarragon is reputed to have a diuretic effect and to stimulate digestion and menstruation. It is also thought to help destroy parasitic worms. The dried roots can be used for toothache. Although tarragon was also known as pellitory or *Bertram* in Hildegard's day, it is probably not the same medicinal herb that she described under this name.

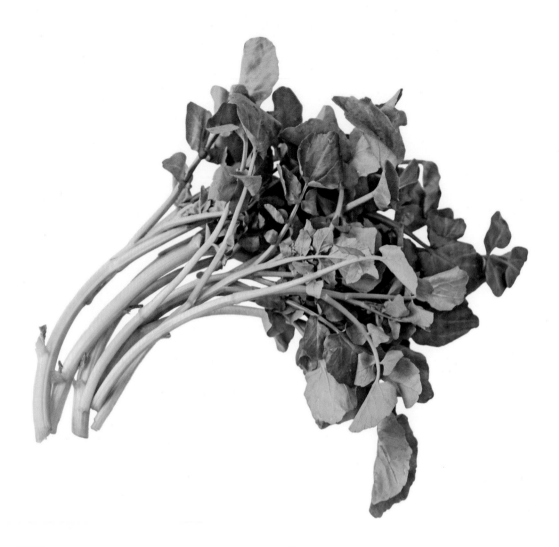

𝔚atercress *(Nasturtium officinale)*

At 12–35 inches (30–90 cm) tall, this perennial bears small, white flowers with yellow stamens held in a terminal pseudo-umbel. The flowers appear in May and last until September. On land, watercress will grow only in meadows with a consistently high level of moisture; otherwise, it is an exclusively aquatic plant that favors clean, flowing water with no risk of freezing in winter. Here, it can form large drifts, spreading along riverbeds via creeping stems attached to the ground by clusters of small roots. Given the right conditions, you can also grow your own watercress. To grow it in a pot, use plenty of compost and place the pot in a tray of water, which should be changed daily. The shoot tips can be harvested toward the end of the winter and in the spring, the leaves all year round as needed. Bear in mind that watercress tastes very peppery during the flowering season. Never pick watercress from polluted water, since the pollutant concentration in the plant will be far too high. Watercress is always used fresh and should be sautéed only briefly in oil. It works well in salads, sauces, and egg dishes and with fried potatoes. Hildegard recommends watercress particularly for people with poor digestion and metabolic disorders.

Water Mint *(Mentha aquatica)*

An herbaceous perennial growing to a height of roughly 30 inches (80 cm), water mint has flowers that appear in dense inflorescences on the shoot tips and, more rarely, in the leaf axils. Water mint grows wild on boggy ground—for example, in wetlands, along streams and rivers, and in ditches. In the garden, it needs shade and plenty of water. It is one of the parent species of peppermint. Its strongly scented leaves and shoot tips are harvested before flowering and added in dried form to meat dishes, soups, sauces, and vegetable dishes. Water mint is especially recommended by Hildegard for digestive, gastric, and gallbladder complaints.

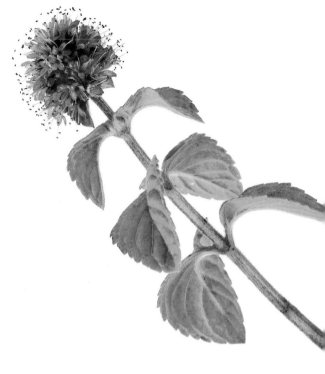

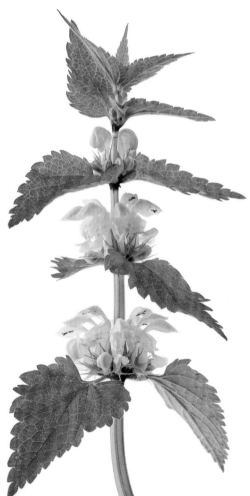

White Dead-Nettle *(Lamium album)*

Well-known plant closely resembling the stinging nettle but with nonstinging leaves (hence the name "dead-nettle"). The white dead-nettle grows to a height of 24 inches (60 cm) and has hairy, serrated, heart-shaped to oval leaves arranged oppositely on hollow, erect stems. The flowers appear from early May in pseudo-whorls on the upper part of the stem. The labiate flowers are pure white. The plant is sown outdoors—or propagated via cuttings—in fall or spring, and it needs sun or semishade and moist, drained soil. The usable parts are the young shoots and leaves harvested prior to flowering, the young plant on its first flowering, and the roots. White dead-nettle is added fresh or dried to soups, sauces, and salads and is recommended in Hildegardian medicine for mood swings and depression.

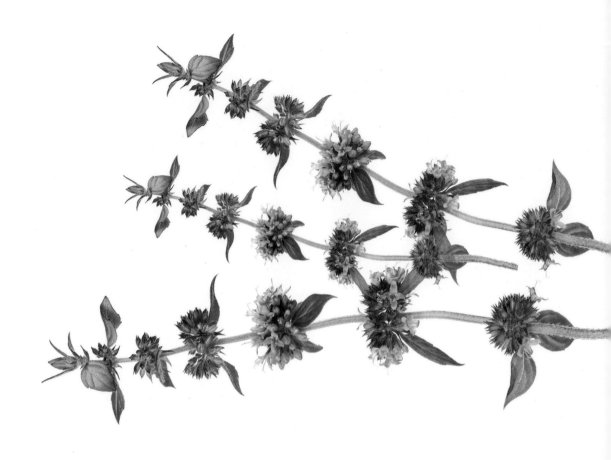

𝔚ild 𝔐int *(Mentha arvensis)*

A small, low-growing herbaceous perennial, wild mint, also known as corn or field mint, grows to a height of 4–12 inches (10–30 cm). Clusters of flowers arranged in false whorls appear along the upper third of the stem and shoots and in the leaf axils from July onward. Grows wild on fallow land and farmland, along waysides and in ditches—provided the soil is moist enough. In the garden, wild mint needs shade and must be kept well watered. Its leaves and young shoots are harvested before flowering and served in dried form with lamb and in salads. They are particularly recommended by Hildegard for stomach and gallbladder complaints.

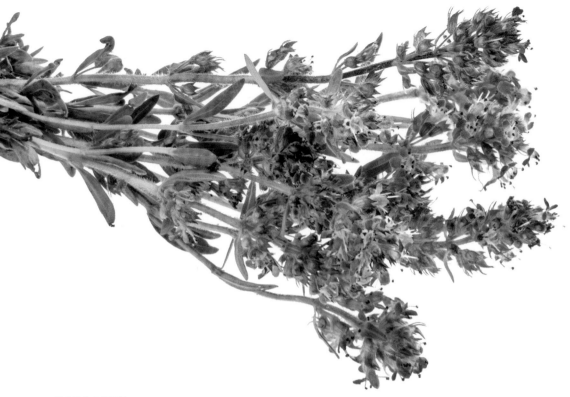

Wild Thyme *(Thymus serpyllum)*

Wild thyme—also known as Breckland thyme or creeping thyme—is a creeping subshrub that grows to a maximum height of 12 inches (30 cm). Its leathery, evergreen oval leaves are intensely fragrant. In the right location, it can also spread over whole areas such as a lawn. With its slightly woody stems, it falls midway between a flowering plant and a woody plant, and it is classified as a subshrub. The small, roughly oval leaflets are arranged oppositely in pairs on the reddish, square stems and give off an intense aroma due to their numerous oil glands. The small pink to violet flowers, which appear in spring, form spherical inflorescences at the tips of the stems. The hermaphrodite flowers ripen in fall into small seeds, allowing the plant to spread by generative propagation and multiplication.

Native to Europe, wild thyme grows naturally on stony ground in upland areas. A winter-hardy plant, it is equally happy in an herb bed or rock garden. It requires little maintenance, but it does need a sunny, dry location. Seedlings are planted outside in early spring and protected with straw in winter. The active substances in the leaves reach their highest concentration before the flowering season, which begins in early summer with the appearance of clusters of pale pink to purple flowers.

The young shoots are dried and used to season meat and vegetable dishes and salads. Hildegard recommends wild thyme for treating skin rashes and purifying the blood. It is important to add the herb during cooking, however, rather than afterward as a condiment. Used in this way, Hildegard claims, it is the key to flawless skin.

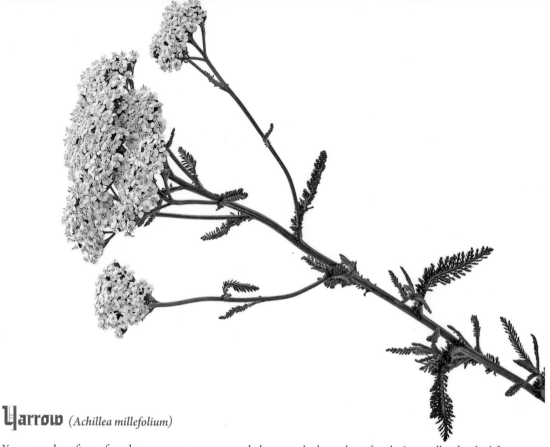

Yarrow *(Achillea millefolium)*

Yarrow—also often referred to as common yarrow—belongs to the huge daisy family. Its small individual flowers are clustered in flat, umbel-like corymbs up to 6 inches (15 cm) wide. These consist of the flower head, measuring just a few millimeters, and the ray florets, which are usually white. The inflorescences are borne on the end of a long stem, which also bears the alternate leaves. Although its scientific name translates as "thousand leaves," this is a false impression created by the pinnate leaves with their countless tooth-edged individual leaflets. Yarrow is widespread in the Northern Hemisphere. It is native to North America, Central America, North Africa, Europe, and North Asia, but it has also been introduced to Africa, Australia, and South America as a result of human migration. Throughout its vast distribution area, it prefers light, warm locations with nutrient-rich soils, such as roadsides, meadows, and pastures. It can be found at altitudes of up to 6,500 feet (2,000 m) or more. Yarrow is also a popular garden plant, with numerous brightly colored varieties now available on the market.

Cultivated yarrow fares particularly well in natural and cottage-style gardens. A low-maintenance plant, it prefers a sunny location with a nutrient-rich but permeable light sandy soil, and it dislikes standing water. Thin soils should be enriched with a little compost, and heavy clayey soils broken up with sand or gravel. The root balls should be well watered before and after planting. To extend the life of this perennial plant, it should be divided every three to four years in spring or fall. Snipping off withered parts and pruning after flowering can help extend the flowering period or stimulate a second bloom.

Yarrow leaves, stems, and flowers were much prized by Hildegard for their many pharmaceutical benefits. Poultices made from the finely chopped leaves are a classic treatment for wounds. The plant can also be used in dried and powdered form, and the leaves and flowers make excellent herbal teas. Last, yarrow is a highly effective aid to recovery after surgery.

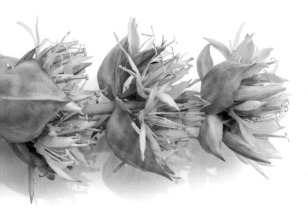

Yellow Gentian *(Gentiana lutea)*

This herbaceous perennial grows to a height of up to 3.3 feet (1 m). It has oppositely arranged leaves that are up to 12 inches (30 cm) long and fused together at the leaf sheaves. The yellow flowers are borne in the leaf axils and appear from June to August. Nowadays, yellow gentian grows wild only in a few upland areas and more commonly in mountainous regions. (Note: In Hildegard's native Germany, this plant now enjoys strict year-round protected status.) In the garden, it needs a sunny location and very thin, dry soil. Hildegard recommends the use of the root, which contains extremely strong, bitter compounds. The dried root is pulverized, and one to three pinches are taken daily with meals for heart and stomach complaints.

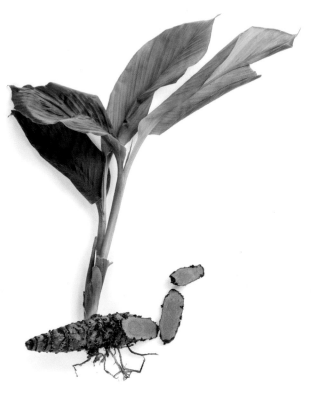

Zedoary *(Curcuma zedoaria)*

Highly valued by Hildegard, zedoary is another name for white turmeric, a spice much lauded nowadays as a "superfood." Growing up to 3.3 feet (1 m) tall, it is native to India but is now grown throughout Southeast Asia, in Japan, and in other locations. The rootstock is harvested for use. Hildegard recommends zedoary boiled in wine for general fortification in case of weakness and for headaches and digestive problems. In powdered form, it is combined with galangal and ginger to make Hildegard's Ginger Mix Powder.

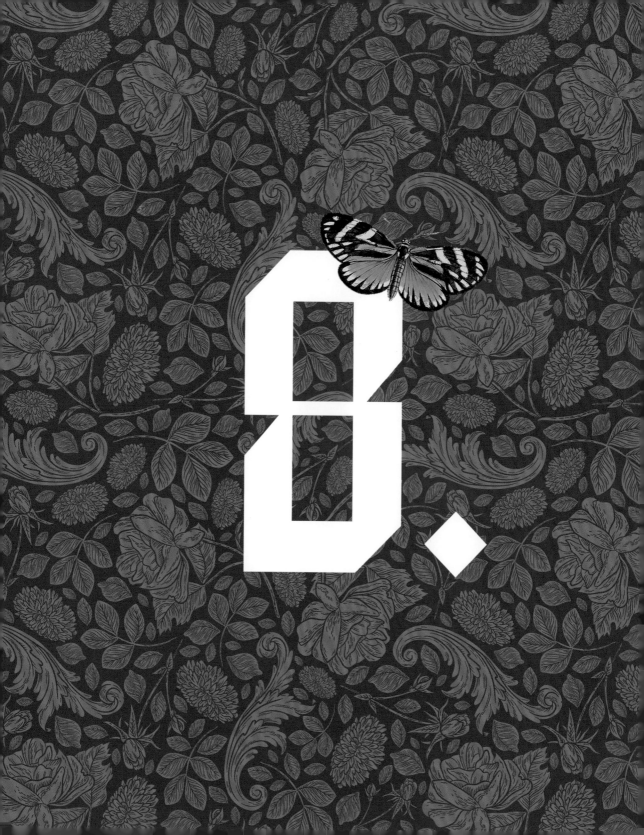

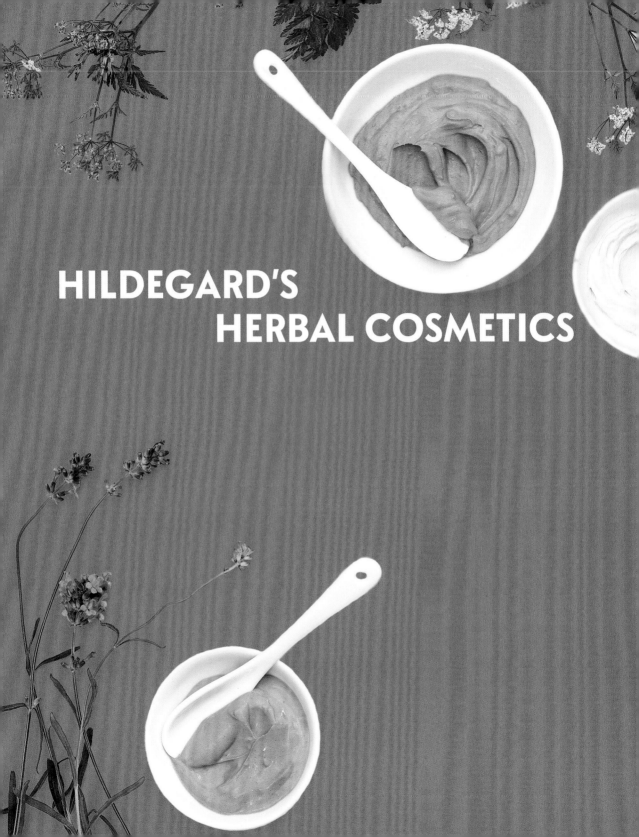

HILDEGARD'S
HERBAL COSMETICS

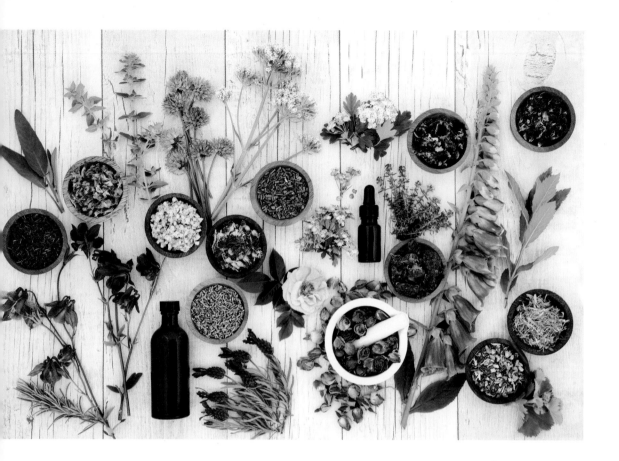

Through her natural medicine, Hildegard of Bingen sought to help people maintain a healthy body on the basis of her holistic approach, which saw physical and mental health as inextricably linked. She stressed in her writings on skin diseases that most are merely a symptom of deeper, underlying conditions and cannot be defeated without thorough cleansing of the gut, but she nevertheless provided many additional tips on how to treat the affected skin directly. As such, her work includes many excursions into the field of cosmetics or beauty care. And the good thing about Hildegardian cosmetics is that they don't call for exotic ingredients; almost all the components available to Hildegard over 850 years ago can still be found relatively easily in our gardens, meadows, and forests.

All the plants used in Hildegardian cosmetics are applied exclusively in the form of infusions, extracts, or pastes. An infusion is prepared simply by pouring boiling water over the herb and leaving it to steep or by boiling it in water for a longer period. Infusions can be applied warm or cold. An extract is made by finely chopping the plant and storing it in oil for a certain time to allow its essential oils and other substances to be absorbed, after which the liquid is filtered off. To make a paste, the plant components are crushed and diluted with water until the right consistency is achieved. None of these preparations require any elaborate equipment, since most of the utensils are common household items.

Scrupulous Hygiene

When preparing cosmetics, scrupulous hygiene must be observed in order to avoid any further skin irritation or rashes. It is therefore important to keep all utensils and containers used in the cosmetic kitchen spotlessly clean. They should be sterilized with boiling water after each use, since anyone preparing natural cosmetics will obviously want to avoid using preservatives. It is a good idea to reserve a suitable pan especially for this purpose. Enamel ones are best for this, since they are easiest to clean. When plant components are boiled, they release a whole range of essential oils, tannins, pigments, and so on into the water that can easily react with the unprotected metal of an ordinary pan. For this reason, you should always use a wooden spoon to stir rather than a metal one.

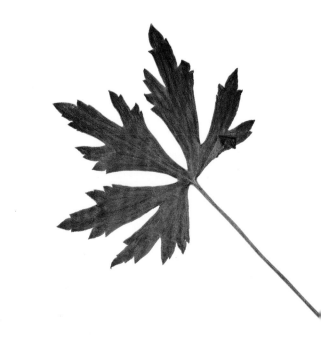

Equipment

The best way to crush the raw materials is to use an old, easily cleaned coffee grinder. A grater is also good for roots and fruits, however. For juicing, the grated plant components are pressed through a clean linen cloth. You will need a funnel to decant the cosmetics into vials, and a measuring beaker is ideal for measuring the required volume of liquid. For basic bath additives—the kind used in hand and foot baths, for example—coarse straining is sufficient and can be done with a simple kitchen strainer. On the other hand, facial and hair tonics, full-body bath additives, and body lotions need a much greater degree of purity and clarity. In this case, an ordinary household strainer is not sufficient; instead, you should use commercially available, unbleached coffee filter papers. This process demands care and patience, however, since the liquids tend to be very viscous and take a long time to pass through the filter—particularly in the case of oil-based extracts. In addition, there is always a risk of tearing the filter paper by squeezing it out too hard. Another good method is to use a muslin diaper or large fabric handkerchief. Alternatively, old nylon tights or stockings can be filled with the plant components like a tea bag; that way, the plant residue can be easily removed after filtration.

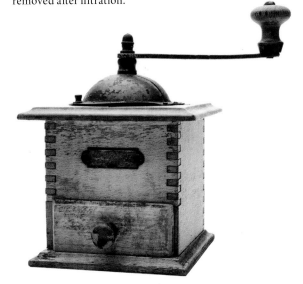

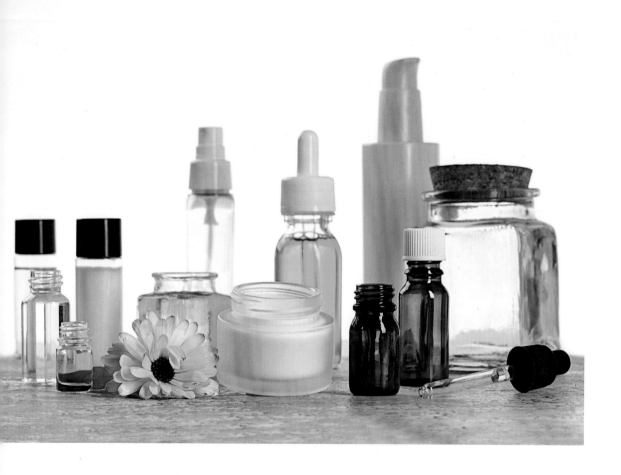

After Preparation

The next step is to decant and store your prepared cosmetics. It's a good idea to start collecting suitable containers in advance—preferably ones that have already had cosmetics in them, such as cream pots, vials, and bottles for tonics, perfume, and bath oils. These should be thoroughly sterilized with boiling water before use, however, in order to remove any residues. It's best not to make overly large quantities, since most homemade cosmetics don't keep very long and should be used within six months at the latest. This is mostly due to the ultraviolet component of sunlight, which causes the products to break down prematurely and lose their efficacy. For this reason, they are best stored in a cool, dark place. In the case of highly perishable products, it is advisable to use dark apothecary bottles; you can ask your local pharmacist if they will sell you a few brown bottles, or you can order some online.

Active Herbal Oils

Ordinary preserving jars are ideal for preparing herbal oils. These can easily be made airtight by sealing them with aluminum foil or plastic wrap. Unused plant ingredients or herbs should first be carefully dried and then stored either in metal tins or jars. The containers should be labeled with the contents and the date of picking. Almost all bioactive cosmetic ingredients lose their efficacy if stored for more than a year.

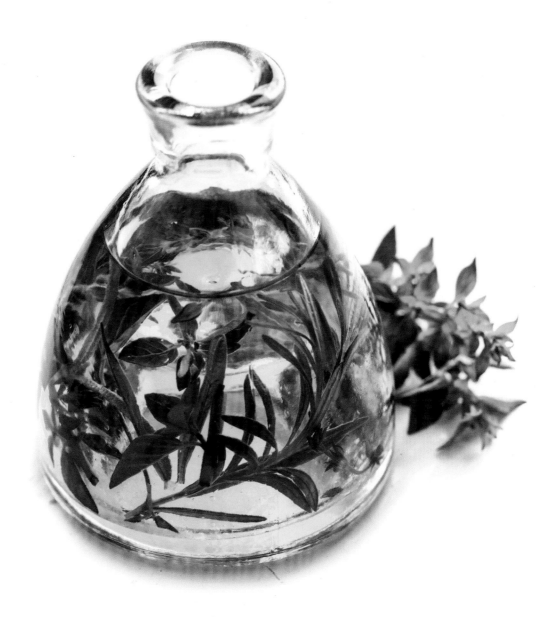

Gentle Compresses

The best way to apply facial compresses is with a small hand towel, since these are just the right size. You can also use an extra-large washcloth, however, and muslin diapers and large fabric handkerchiefs make other good alternatives. When applying the compresses, make sure they are well moistened, and keep dampening them as necessary. For the area around the eyes, it is best to use cotton balls or extra-soft tissues. Coarse face masks can be applied with your hands, but runnier ones will need a brush. Ideally, you should use a special cosmetic brush for this, but if you don't have one or prefer not to use one, you can use a paintbrush instead. Be sure to keep it exclusively for this purpose, however, and rinse it out with hot water after each use. When applying face masks and intensive hair treatments, always use a plastic shower cap to protect your hair or face respectively.

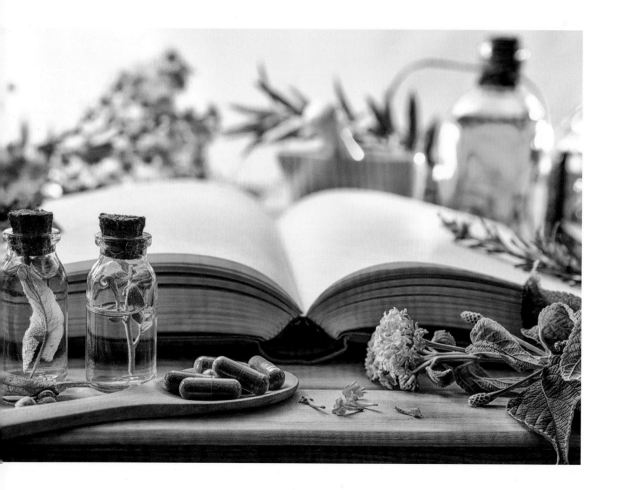

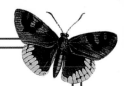

Hildegardian Cosmetics

The main plants and their uses in Hildegard's cosmetic kitchen are described in the table below. The left column lists the relevant plants, the center column describes the preparation method, and the right column details the type of application.

PLANT	PREPARATION	APPLICATION
Alder	Leaf infusion	Bath additive
Apple	Paste	Face mask
Aquilegia (columbine)	Infusion	Facial toner
Arnica	Flower infusion	Steam bath / hair conditioner
Basil	Infusion	Mouthwash
Beans	Paste	Face mask
Birch	Leaf infusion	Facial toner / hair conditioner / pedicure
Boxwood	Ointment	Ointment for wounds/scabs
Boxwood	Infusion	Hair color
Burdock	Root infusion	Hair care
Cabbage	Paste	Face mask
Calendula	Ointment	Ointment for skin irritations
Calendula	Infusion	Facial toner
Celandine	Infusion	Facial care / hair conditioner
Celery	Infusion	Facial toner
Centaury	Infusion	Facial compress
Chamomile	Infusion	Skin care / bath additive
Coltsfoot	Infusion	Skin care / hair care / steam bath
Comfrey	Root infusion	Facial toner / skin lotion

PLANT	PREPARATION	APPLICATION
Cowslip	Infusion	Bath additive
Cucumber	Paste	Face mask
Elder	Flower infusion	Facial toner / steam bath
Elecampane	Root infusion	Facial toner
Fennel	Infusion	Facial toner / steam bath
Garlic	Raw clove	Treatment for corns
Hawthorn	Infusion	Hair tonic / steam bath
Horse chestnut	Paste	Paste for treating cellulitis
Horseradish	Infusion	Facial care
Horsetail	Infusion	Facial care / hair conditioner
Ivy	Infusion	Infusion for skin eczema / cellulitis
Ivy	Leaf paste	Paste for treating corns
Lavender	Flower infusion	Facial toner / hair tonic / bath additive
Lavender	Oil extract	Body lotion
Lemon balm	Infusion	Steam bath / bath additive
Lettuce	Extract	Face mask
Lovage	Infusion	Bath additive / foot bath
Lily	Infusion	Facial toner
Linden	Flower infusion	Facial toner / hair tonic / steam bath / bath additive
Mallow	Extract	Facial toner
Marshmallow	Ointment	Face mask
Oak	Bark infusion	Bath additive
Onion	Infusion	Hair tonic

PLANT	PREPARATION	APPLICATION
Parsley	Infusion	Skin tonic
Peach	Paste	Face mask
Peach	Leaf infusion	Hair tonic
Pear	Halved fruit	Facial massage
Peppermint	Infusion	Steam bath
Peppermint	Extract	Body oil
Pine	Ointment	Eye care ointment
Quince	Seed paste	Hair gel
Ribwort plantain	Infusion	Facial compress
Rose	Infusion	Facial toner / hair tonic / bath additive
Rose	Oil extract	Body lotion
Rosemary	Infusion	Facial toner / hair tonic
Sage	Infusion	Hair conditioner / bath additive
Savory	Infusion	Facial toner
Stinging nettle	Infusion	Hair tonic / hair conditioner
Stinging nettle	Extract	Skin lotion
Saint-John's-wort	Infusion/extract	Face pack
Strawberries	Paste	Face mask
Thyme	Infusion	Bath additive
Violet	Ointment	Skin care
Watercress	Infusion	Facial care
Willow	Leaf infusion	Hair tonic
Yarrow	Infusion	Face pack

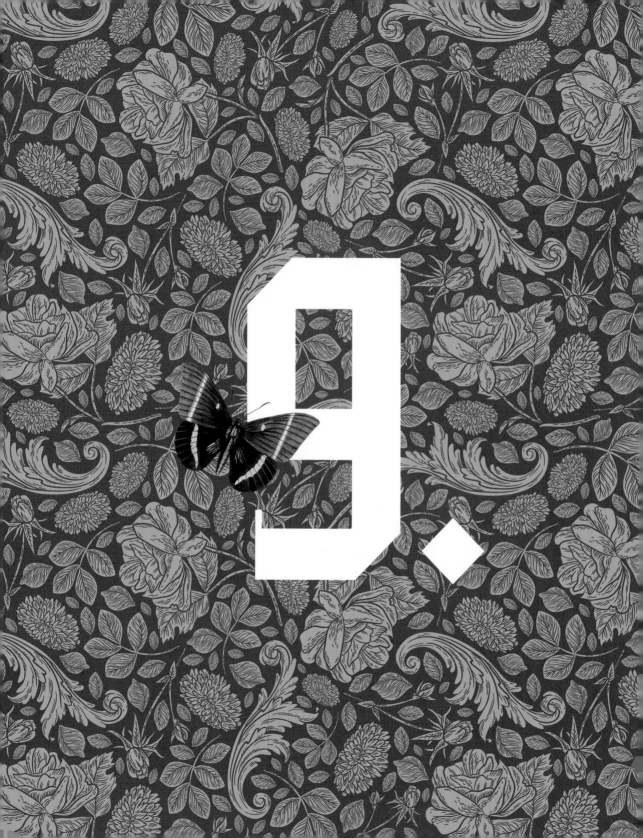

9.

HILDEGARD OF BINGEN AND GEMSTONES

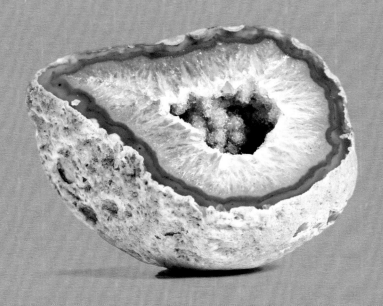

In her book *Scivias*, Hildegard of Bingen had the following to say about gemstones: "Each stone contains fire. The infernal host is repelled by precious stones and hates them, for they remind it of its origin in the fire in which the fallen angels now serve their punishment."

was jasper, the second sapphire, the third agate, the fourth emerald" (Revelation 21:19). A further biblical example of the veneration of gemstones is the fact that the high priest—the chief religious functionary in the temple—wore a breastplate adorned with jewels, each bearing the name of one of the twelve tribes of Israel.

The Power of Gemstones

The use of all kinds of gemstones in prehistoric and ancient healing was an integral part of the contemporaneous medical art. Written records in the ancient Indian language of Sanskrit describing the power of crystals can be traced back as far as 400 BCE. Archeological finds from India, ancient Egypt, and ancient Greece likewise testify to the importance of crystals in medicine. The special role of gemstones and the reverence in which they were held are also reflected in the Bible. Of the city of Jerusalem, described as "coming down out of heaven from God" after "the first heaven and the first earth had passed away," the Bible says: "The foundations of the city walls were decorated with every kind of precious stone. The first foundation

Hildegard's Healing Stones

In her works *Physica* and *Causae et Curae*, Hildegard wrote about the possible applications and effect of gemstones in natural medicine. Although she cannot have known anything about the geological processes involved in the stones' formation, she gives an accurate description here of the different forms of crystal growth. With their uniform exterior and inherently high degree of organization, they differ markedly from the rest of nature, which appears to us as largely chaotic. Both primary minerals (such as crystals from the earth's interior or escaping lava) and secondary minerals (formed on the earth's surface due to the impact of heat, air, and water) are shaped by the perfect harmony and unity of the atoms that go into making up a crystal. It

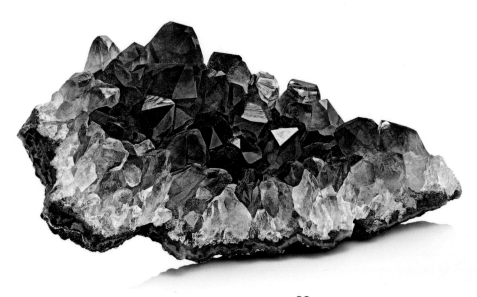

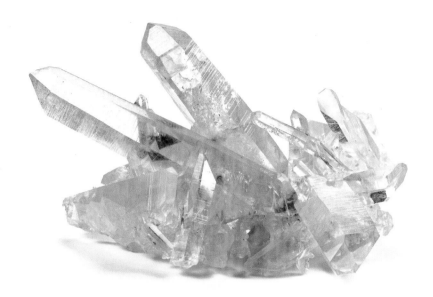

was therefore natural in medieval times to see in this the ordering hand of God. According to Hildegard: "The heavenly energies of Creation fused with fragments of matter and turned them into carriers of energy which transmit useful and healing energies. Each precious stone unlocks certain parts of our soul like a key. The soul and the stone know each other and have a mutually energizing effect. This leads to healing processes in the body." Fever, for example, should be treated with topaz. Someone with "falling sickness" (epilepsy) should "place an agate stone in water for three days, take it out on the fourth, heat it gently, and use it to cook all his food; he should do this for ten moons, and he will be cured—unless it be not God's will." Hildegard's writings on gemstones still pose many riddles for scholars today, however. There is now a general consensus, for example, that numerous passages were changed in a subsequent revision, particularly those describing the stones' magic powers. And it remains ultimately unclear whether other parts of her work are authentic or might have been added much later.

Gemstone Medicine Today

To this day, there are alternative medical techniques that advocate the use of gemstones to cure diseases. Within traditional medicine, attitudes toward gemstone therapy range from critical to skeptical at best, but most practitioners reject it altogether. Even so, there are many people who do believe in the medicinal properties of gemstones. They argue that there are vibrations within the human body just as there are in gemstones, and that these can influence each other. The key to healing a disease, therefore, is to select the right stone with the right vibrations. Advocates of gemstone therapy essentially believe that each stone has its own curative effect. As with all phenomena that cannot be adequately explained by science, there are also various currents of thought within gemstone medicine. Like Hildegard, gemstone therapists attribute different medicinal effects to different stones. Most also have personal favorites, however—such as quartz crystal, for instance—that they credit with the greatest healing power.

There are several methods of gemstone application. The most common, which Hildegard also regards as most important, is to place a stone on the skin above the affected organ. For long-term therapies, the stone can be kept in place by wearing it on a chain or bracelet, for example. Please note however that this method cannot be used on young children, for whom necklaces in particular can pose fatal risks. In their case, it is better to put the stone in a small bag and place it inside their pillow. In addition to these methods, there are also recipes for preparing healing waters or powders from certain gemstones. All stones should be washed in cold water before use, as Hildegard herself advised. She appears keen to make the point—also supported by gemstone therapists—that no one should rely exclusively on stones to cure them, particularly in the case of serious organic illnesses. Gemstone medicine should only ever be used as a complement to expert medical treatment.

Science or Occultism?

In contrast to the generally accepted, logical principles of Hildegard's nutritional therapy, which in many cases anticipated the scientific discoveries of modern medicine and nutritional research, her gemstone medicine is not uncontroversial today. The reason for this is the appropriation of Hildegard herself, as an iconic female figure of the European medieval period, by esoteric circles and communities into whose worldview Hildegard's gemstone therapy, taken out of context, seems to fit perfectly. The Association of Christian Naturopaths in Germany, for example, considers the use of gemstones for medicinal purposes dangerous "not because of any problem with the stones themselves, but because esoteric methods are used to exploit the physical and mental vulnerability of the sick and, instead of delivering a proven naturopathic treatment method, presents them with a substitute that is often propagated with seductive promises but doesn't stand up to scrutiny and can lead to a spiritual bondage to the occult." This is a general problem of our modern age, however, and cannot diminish the outstanding achievement of Hildegard, who saw the harmony of gemstones as proof of God's work: "O power of eternity, who have ordered all things in your heart: by your word all things are created as you have willed."

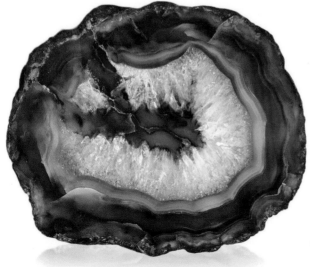

Hildegard's Gemstone Medicine

The following stones are used in Hildegardian gemstone medicine:

NAME	COLOR	FIELD OF APPLICATION
Agate	Semitransparent to opaque, in various shades of gray	Epilepsy, insect bites
Amethyst	Transparent violet	Skin complaints, insect infestation
Beryl	Transparent colorless, pale green, gray, or pink	Nervous disorders
Carnelian	Transparent, in shades of red	Nosebleeds
Chalcedony	Semitransparent to opaque, blue, yellow, grayish red, or white	Weakness
Chrysolite	Various shades of green	Fever, heart problems
Chrysoprase	Transparent to opaque in various shades of green	Epilepsy, gout
Diamond	Transparent, usually colorless, but also yellowish to black	Liver complaints, alcoholism, gout, stroke
Emerald	Transparent green	Epilepsy, heart problems, stomach ailments, ulcers, headache
Hyacinth	Transparent red brown	Fever, eye problems
Jasper	Semitransparent to opaque, blue, brown, yellow, greenish red, or black	Ear problems, gout, colds
Onyx	Black or mottled white	Eye problems, fever, heart problems, stomach ailments
Quartz crystal	Transparent colorless, occasionally brownish to black	Eye problems, thyroid disorders, heart problems, stomach ailments
Ruby	Transparent red	Gout, fever, headache
Sapphire	Transparent blue	Eye problems, heart problems, gastric complaints, ulcers, headache
Sard	Brownish	Ear problems, fever, liver complaints
Sardonyx	Brown and white banded	Intellectual weakness
Topaz	Semitransparent blue, brown, yellow, green, or white	Eye problems, fever

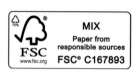